PHARMACOLOGY IN DRUG DISCOVERY

UNDERSTANDING DRUG RESPONSE

T0383230

PHARMACOLOGY IN DRUG DISCOVERY

UNDERSTANDING DRUG RESPONSE

TERRY P. KENAKIN, PhD

*Department of Pharmacology, University of North Carolina School of Medicine,
Chapel Hill, NC, USA*

AMSTERDAM • BOSTON • HEIDELBERG • LONDON • NEW YORK • OXFORD
PARIS • SAN DIEGO • SAN FRANCISCO • SINGAPORE • SYDNEY • TOKYO

Academic Press is an imprint of Elsevier

Academic Press is an imprint of Elsevier
32 Jamestown Road, London NW1 7BY, UK
225 Wyman Street, Waltham, MA 02451, USA
525 B Street, Suite 1800, San Diego, CA 92101-4495, USA

First edition 2012

British Library Cataloguing-in-Publication Data
A catalogue record for this book is available from the British Library

Library of Congress Cataloging-in-Publication Data
A catalog record for this book is available from the Library of Congress

ISBN : 978-0-12-384856-7

For information on all Academic Press publications
visit our website at elsevierdirect.com

Typeset by MPS Limited, A Macmillan Company, Chennai, India
www.macmillansolutions.com

Printed and bound by CPI Group (UK) Ltd, Croydon, CR0 4YY

Transferred to digital print 2012

As Always . . . for Debbie

Contents

Foreword

In the scheme of science, pharmacology is a relatively new scientific discipline branching off, in the last century, from the older more established science of physiology. The term can have a range of meanings from the study of drug action to the design of new drugs. These nuances in terminology are associated with the way pharmacology is presented and taught. To a medical student, pharmacology may mean the properties of therapeutic drugs and the study of how they are used in therapy (i.e., therapeutics). To a researcher it may mean the study of drug mechanism of action. To a scientist working in drug discovery, it may mean the application of medicinal chemistry to modify physiology for therapeutic benefit.

This text is designed to introduce all students who may need to interpret a change in physiology induced by a chemical substance. Physiological systems customize chemical signal input to their own needs; thus the same drug can have different effects in different physiological systems. Pharmacology is unique in that it furnishes the tools to analyze these different behaviors and trace them to their root cause, i.e., the molecular mechanism of action. This enables predictions of drug behavior to be made in all systems, an invaluable tool for drug discovery since almost all drugs are developed in test systems far removed from the therapeutic one. This text should enable the reader to interpret drug dose—response data and make mechanistic inferences at the molecular level.

Terry Kenakin Ph.D.
Research Triangle Park, 2011

Acknowledgements

I wish specifically to thank Kristine Jones and April Graham of Elsevier for patient support of this project and so very much help. I also wish to thank Dr. Angela Finch, University of Sydney, for valuable comments and guidance. The excellent artwork of Candy Webster was indispensable in the production of this book and I wish to thank her for her wonderful efforts. I am indebted to GlaxoSmithKline for support during the preparation of this book and to the University of North Carolina School of Medicine for giving me the means to explore pharmacology and apply it to drug discovery. Finally, I am very grateful to my wife and family for boundless patience during the writing of this book.

1

Pharmacology: The Chemical Control of Physiology

By the end of this chapter the reader should be able to understand how drug response is quantified by the use of dose–response curves, the way in which different tissues process drug stimulus to provide tissue response and what qualifies a drug to be classified either as an agonist or antagonist.

PHARMACOLOGY AND CELLULAR DRUG RESPONSE

Pharmacology (from the Greek φαρμακον, pharmakon, "drug" and -λογία, -logia, the study of) concerns drug action on physiological systems (physiology from the Greek φύσις, physis, "nature, origin" and -λογία, -logia is the study of the mechanical, physical and biochemical functions of living organisms). With regard to the application of pharmacology to the discovery of drugs for therapeutic benefit, the main focus of pharmacological theories, procedures and mechanisms relates to the *chemical control of physiological processes*. Insofar as the understanding of these physiological processes benefits the pharmacologic pursuit of drugs, pharmacology and physiology are intimately related. However, it will also be seen that complete understanding of the physiologic processes involved is *not* a prerequisite to the effective use of pharmacology in the drug discovery process. In fact, often an operational approach is utilized whereby the complexity of the physiology is represented by simple surrogate mathematical functions.

A unique feature of pharmacology is that the effect of the drug is often observed indirectly, that is, while the drug affects a select biochemical process in the cell, the outcome to an observer is an overall change in the state of the whole organism, and this is often the result of multiple interacting cellular processes. A major aim of pharmacology is to define the molecular events in initiating drug effects, since these define the action of drugs in all systems. If quantified correctly, this information can be used to predict drug effect at the pharmacological target in all systems including therapeutic one(s). At this point, it is useful to define what is meant by pharmacological target.

NEW TERMINOLOGY

The following new terms will be introduced in this chapter:

- **Affinity**: The propensity of a drug molecule to associate closely with a drug target.
- **Agonists**: Drugs that produce an observable change in the state of a physiological system.
- **Antagonists**: Drugs that may not produce a direct effect, but do interfere with the production of cellular response to an agonist.
- **Dose–response curve**: The relationship between doses (if the drug is used *in vivo*) or concentrations (if used *in vitro*) of a drug and pharmacologic effect.
- **Drug target**: The protein (or in some cases DNA, mRNA) to which a drug binds to elicit whatever pharmacologic effect it will produce. These proteins can be seven transmembrane (or one transmembrane) receptors, enzymes, nuclear receptors, ion channels or transport proteins.
- **EC_{50}**: Concentration of agonist producing half the maximal response to the same agonist; usually expressed for calculation and statistical manipulation as the pEC_{50},

negative logarithm of the molar concentration producing 50% response.
- **Efficacy**: The change in state of the drug target upon binding of a drug.
- **Efficiency of target coupling**: The relationship between the net quanta of activation given to a cell and the number of drug targets available for activation.
- **Full agonists**: Agonists that produce the full maximal response that the system can produce.
- **Null method**: The comparison of equiactive concentrations (or doses) of drug to cancel the cell-based processing of drug response. The assumption is that equal responses to a given agonist are processed in an identical manner by the cell.
- **Partial agonists**: Agonists that produce a maximal response that is of lower magnitude than the maximal response that the system can produce to maximal stimulation.
- **pEC_{50}**: The negative logarithm of EC_{50} values. For arithmetic and/or statistical manipulation, numbers must be normally distributed. This is true only of pEC_{50}s, not of EC_{50}s; thus all averages, estimates or error and statistical procedures must use pEC_{50}.
- **Potency**: The concentration (usually molar) of drug needed to produce a defined response or effect.
- **Target density**: The concentration of drug targets at the site of activation, i.e., on the cell surface for receptors.

PHARMACOLOGICAL TARGETS

The term "pharmacological target" refers to the biochemical entity to which the drug first binds in the body to elicit its effect. There are a number of such entities targeted by drug molecules. In general, they can be proteins such as receptors, enzymes, transporters, ion channels, or genetic material such as DNA. The prerequisite for pharmacologic targets is that they have the ability to discern differences in electronic structure minute enough to be present in small drug-like molecules; in this regard the most predominant targets for drugs are protein in nature. Proteins have the tertiary three-dimensional structure necessary for detailed definition of the electronic forces involved in small molecule binding. Signals are initiated through complementary binding of drug molecules to protein conformations that have a physiological purpose in the cell. The act of these molecules binding to the protein will change it, and with that change a pharmacologic effect will occur.

At this point, it is worth considering the beginning and end processes. The first process is the drug binding to the target. The result(s) of this process are totally dependent on the affinity and efficacy of the drug. These are drug parameters unique to its chemical structure. In pharmacologic terms, this is the most important effect, since it occurs in each and every tissue and organ possessing the target. Therefore, characterization of this event enables a general quantification of drug-target activity to be made in the test system, which will also be true for all systems including the therapeutic one. Therefore, *the characterization of affinity and efficacy become the primary aim of pharmacologic analysis*. However, it can be seen that the various (and variable) biochemical reactions linking the target to cellular response intervene, thereby causing a tissue-dependent abstraction of the link between affinity and efficacy and observed cellular potency. The magnitude of this abstraction depends upon the number of responding target units and the efficiency of target coupling.

The major protein target classes are membrane receptors, enzymes, ion channels and transporter proteins. Of these, the most prominent drug targets are receptors. While there are a number of types of receptor, one of the most important from the standpoint of therapeutic drug targets is seven transmembrane receptors (7TMRs). These are so-called because they span the cell membrane seven times to form complex recognition domains both outside and inside the cell. These proteins are capable of recognizing chemicals such as hormones and neurotransmitters present in the extracellular space, and transmit signals from these to the cell interior. Due to the fact that these are on the cell surface and thus exposed to the extracellular space, these entities were the subject of experiments that originally defined the receptor concept (see Box 1.1 for history).

Historically, while the actual physical nature of receptors was unknown, it was realized that a distinct entity on the cell surface allows cells to recognize drugs and read the chemical information encoded in them. Early concepts of receptors likened them to locks with drugs as keys (i.e., as stated by the biologist Paul Ehrlich: "... *substances can only be anchored at any particular part of the organism if they fit into the molecule of the recipient complex like a piece of mosaic finds its place in a pattern...*"). The main value of receptors is that they put order into the previously disordered world of physiology. For example, it has been observed that the hormone epinephrine produces a wealth of dissimilar physiological responses such as bronchiole muscle relaxation, cardiac muscle positive inotropy, chronotropy and lusitropy, melatonin synthesis, pancreatic, lacrimal and salivary gland secretion, decreased stomach motility, urinary bladder muscle relaxation, skeletal muscle tremor and vascular relaxation. The understanding of how such a vast array of biological responses could be mediated by a single hormone is difficult until it is realized that these processes are all mediated by the interaction of epinephrine with a single receptor protein, in this case

BOX 1.1

THE EVOLUTION OF THE RECEPTOR CONCEPT IN PHARMACOLOGY

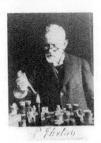

Numerous physiologists and pharmacologists contributed to the concept of "receptor" as minimal recognition units for chemicals in cells. Paul Ehrlich (1854–1915) studied dyes and bacteria and determined that there are "chemoreceptors" (he proposed a collection of "amboreceptors," "triceptors" and "polyceptors") on parasites, cancer cells and microorganisms that could be exploited therapeutically.

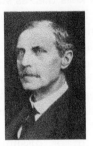

John Newport Langley (1852–1926), as Chair of the Physiology Department in Cambridge, studied the drugs jaborandi (containing the alkaloid pilocarpine) and atropine. He concluded that receptors were "switches" that received and generated signals and that these switches could be activated or blocked by specific molecules.

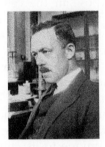

A. J. Clark (1885–1941), who could be considered the father of modern receptor pharmacology, was one of the first to suggest from studies of acetylcholine and atropine that a unimolecular interaction occurs between a drug and a "substance on the cell." As stated by Clark: "... it is impossible to explain the remarkable effects observed except by assuming that drugs unite with receptors of a highly specific pattern..."

the β-adrenoceptor. Thus, when this receptor is present on the surface of any given cell it will respond to epinephrine, and the nature of that response will be determined by the encoding of the receptor excitation produced by epinephrine to the cytosolic biochemical cascades controlling cellular function. In a conceptual sense, the term "receptor" can refer to any single biological entity that responds to drugs (i.e., enzymes, ion channels, transport proteins, DNA and structures in the nucleus). This information is transmitted through changes in protein shape (conformation) i.e., the drug does not enter the cell nor does the receptor change the nature of the drug (as an enzyme would).

Pharmacologic targets can be used to modify physiological processes. Specifically, chemicals can be used to cause activation, blockade or modulation of protein receptors and ion channel targets. For enzymes and transporter proteins the main drug effect is inhibition of ongoing basal activity of these targets (Chapter 6 discusses these targets in detail). Another difference between these target classes is location; while receptors, ion channels and transporter proteins are usually found on the cell surface (exposed to the extracellular space), enzymes are most often found in the cytosol of the cell (drugs must enter the cell to act on enzymes). Exceptions to this general rule are nuclear receptors which reside in the cell nucleus. Finally, it should be recognized that there are other drug targets present in the cell, such as DNA, and that chemicals can have physical effects (i.e., membrane stabilization) that can change cellular function.

Pharmacologic effects on cells can include a wide variety of outcomes, from changes in the mechanical function of cells (i.e., cardiac contractility, contraction of bronchiole smooth muscle), biochemical metabolic effects (levels of second messengers such as calcium ion or cyclic AMP) and modulation of basal activity (level of catalytic degradation of cyclic AMP by enzymes such as phosphodiesterase, rate of uptake of neuroamines such as norepinephrine and serotonin).

It is worth considering the process of target choice in the drug discovery process. Specifically, effective prosecution of any drug target requires a minimal effort in resources and time (perhaps 1 to 2 years per target), thus it can be seen how an incorrect choice of target could lead to a serious dissimulation in the drug discovery process. While there are considerations in target choice, such as target tractability (how difficult it is to produce a molecule to alter the behavior of the target), one of the most important factors is a strong association with the disease that is being treated. It has been estimated that there are approximately 600 to 1500 possible drug targets that may be valid to pursue for therapy. These are made up of genes that are known to be associated with diseases and that also code for protein that may be modified through binding to a small molecule.[1] No discovery program could pursue a number of genes close to the number available, making target validation a very important step in the process. Table 1.1 shows some of the factors involved in the process of target validation, with particular reference to the problem of HIV-1 viral entry to cause Acquired Immune Deficiency Syndrome (AIDS). As a preface to the discussion of cellular drug effect, it is useful to consider the major pharmacological tool used to quantify it, namely, the dose—response curve.

DOSE—RESPONSE CURVES

A characteristic feature of drugs acting on a specific target in a physiological system is that there will be a graded increase in response with an increase in drug concentration (dose). If drug effect can be observed directly, then the magnitude of effect can be displayed as a function of drug concentration in the form of a dose—response curve. For example, epinephrine is known to cause increased heart rate in humans; Fig. 1.1 shows how increasing doses of epinephrine produce increases in heart rate. The curve-defining dose and resulting observed response can be used as shorthand to characterize the effect of the drug in the system. This relationship can then be used to predict what any dose of the drug will do in the system, in the form of an empirically derived line joining the observed data points. Figure 1.2 shows the increased heart rate as a function of epinephrine concentration. The lines joining the data points infer that there is a continuous relationship between epinephrine dose and heart rate. Such an empirical

TABLE 1.1   Factors Relevant to Target Validation with Reference to AIDS

Factor	CCR5 in AIDS	Reference
• Target is linked to sensitivity to disease	• CCR5 receptors must be present on cell surface for HIV-1 infection	[2,3]
• Cell level of target alters sensitivity and course of disease	• Down-regulation of CCR5 leads to resistance to HIV-1 infection	[4]
	• Genetically high levels of CCR5 lead to rapid progression to AIDS	[5]
• Interference with target will not lead to harm	• CCR5 knockout mouse[1] lacks the receptor but is otherwise healthy	[6]
• Ligands for target interfere with disease	• CCR5 interaction with chemokines interfere with HIV-1 infection	[7–11]
	• Patients with high circulating levels of chemokine have retarded progression to AIDS	[12,13]
• Specific genetic association	• Δ32 deletion in CCR5 gene leads to lack of receptor expression and complete resistance to AIDS	[14–18]

[1]Genetically altered mouse that does not naturally express the CCR5 receptor.

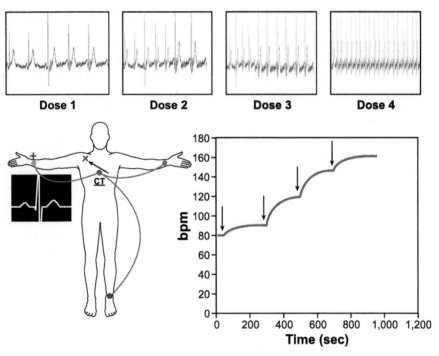

FIGURE 1.1   Dose–response curve for epinephrine given to a human at increasing doses. The heart rate is obtained from non-invasive EKG leads. It can be seen that there is a relationship between heart rate and increasing dose of epinephrine.

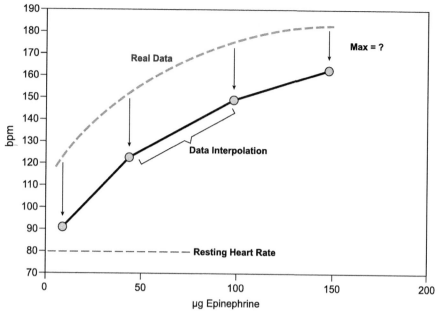

FIGURE 1.2 Empirically-determined dose–response curve for data shown in Fig. 1.1. Real data points joined by straight lines enable responses to doses between 8 μg and 144 μg to be predicted. While the basal activity of the system is known (patient's resting heart rate = 80 bpm), the true maximum of the curve is unknown.

relationship can allow interpolation of values, but the predictions must be bounded by real data to do so. Usually the basal activity of the system is known (i.e., in the case of the example, the patient had a resting heart rate of 80 bpm). Dose–response relationships are characterized by three parameters; a threshold, slope and maximum. In the example shown in Fig. 1.2, the threshold can be inferred from the increase from 80 bpm and the slope from the existing real data points. The maximum response can be problematic since, unless it can be defined by real data, it must be projected from the existing data; this will be discussed in more detail in the following consideration of dose–response relationships. In this case, as in many pharmacological cases, there are safety issues for experimentally determining the maximal heart rate increase to epinephrine (i.e., a fatal arrhythmia could ensue). For this reason, dose–response data

is often used to apply mathematical models that can fully define the dose–response relationship. As a preface to this discussion, it is useful to consider what a dose–response relationship represents in a physiological system.

Figure 1.3 shows a typical dose–response curve. Considering a living cell as an idling engine, there is a basal level of activity that is an ambient baseline for the dose–response curve; an analogy could be that cellular metabolism is a faucet of water filling a container with a hole in it. If the level of the water in the container is the cellular effect, then an input can be sub-threshold if the rate of exit of the water keeps the level low (see Fig. 1.3). As the stimulus to the cell increases (increased flow of water into the container) the level rises visibly, and this can be viewed as the cellular response to the drug. At some point, a maximum will be attained whereby the system can

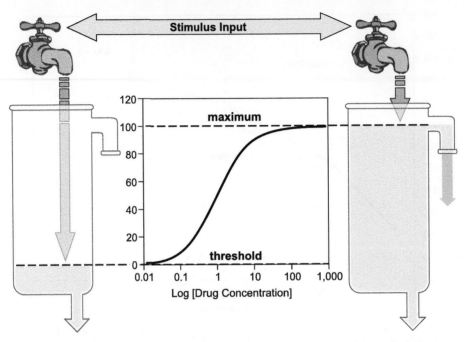

FIGURE 1.3 Schematic of a cell process described by a dose—response curve. The stimulus input is the amount of fluid entering the vessel from the spigot; the level of fluid in the vessel is the cellular response. It is assumed that the cell has a basal activity, given by a low level of fluid entry into the vessel. The level of the fluid at this point describes the basal activity of the cell. As a drug increases the stimulus to the system (increases fluid entry), the level of the fluid rises (cellular response increases). At some point, the level exceeds the limits of the vessel and escapes through the overflow; this represents the maximal capability of the cell to increase activity.

return no further response to a stimulus. These cellular maxima can be dictated by the physiological or mechanical properties of the cell (saturation of a biochemical process or attainment of a maximal mechanical contraction). This can be modeled as an overflow valve to prevent the level of water from going above a certain level (Fig. 1.3). Thus, a window of response for the cell exists between the threshold and maximum where a drug may change cellular effect, and the strength of that effect will be linked to the concentration of the drug by a quantifiable function. This function is visualized as a dose—response curve. A useful expedient is to express the dosage on a logarithmic scale. This allows a wide range of doses to be shown

concisely and the maximum to be more easily observed. These details will be discussed more fully in the section on the Langmuir adsorption isotherm. Figure 1.4 shows the dose—response relationship given in Fig. 1.1 and Fig. 1.2 on a logarithmic scale fit with a mathematical function. The maximum response in this case was obtained from historical data suggesting that a maximal heart rate of 220 bpm is common for human heart muscle. The nature of various mathematical fitting functions for dose—response data will be discussed further in Chapter 2.

It is worth mentioning at this point how the design of pharmacologic experiments is based on an independent variable (drug

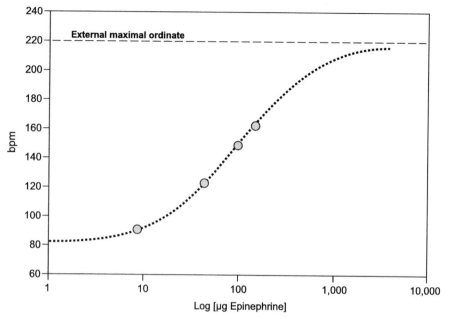

FIGURE 1.4 Data from Fig. 1.2 fit to a semi-logarithmic sigmoidal mathematical function that covers a larger range of doses. The maximal heart rate is taken from historical data (220 bpm for normal healthy humans).

concentration) being put into an organ system to yield a dependent variable (drug response); on the basis of the magnitude of the dependent variable, drugs are characterized in terms of potency and efficacy. This system is based on the tacit assumption that the value of the independent variable is accurately known. If the concentration of drug at the target is not known accurately, then all subsequent estimates of drug activity (which go on to be ascribed to be characteristics of the drug) are also wrong. Therefore, it is imperative that exemplary care be taken to accurately determine the value of drug concentration interacting with the target. This is exceptionally difficult *in vivo*, hence an entire discipline around this problem has evolved in the form of **pharmacokinetics**. This will be dealt with explicitly in Chapters 7 and 8. Pharmacology also utilizes *in vitro* experimentation in which tissues are incubated in media mimicking true physiology in chambers of constant volume, to obviate variance in drug concentration and thus accurately link concentration to drug activity. This technology was first introduced into pharmacology by pioneers such as Magnus at the turn of the century (see Box 1.2).

On a semi-logarithmic scale, dose–response curves are characteristically sigmoidal in shape (i.e., see Fig. 1.4). The location parameters of such curves denote the **potency** of the drug. If the dose–response curve is obtained *in vivo*, then the EC_{50} will be a measure such as mg/kg body weight. If the experiment is done *in vitro*, then a molar potency can be obtained. For *in vitro* experiments a convenient parameter to numerically quantify potency is to report the pEC_{50} of the curve, literally the negative logarithm of the molar concentration of the drug that produces half the maximal response to the drug (see Fig. 1.5A). The pEC_{50} is the correct form to use for EC_{50} manipulation

BOX 1.2

ISOLATED TISSUE PHARMACOLOGY

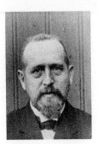

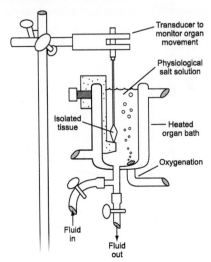

Rudolf Magnus (1873–1927) was a German pharmacologist who became the first Professor of Pharmacology at the University of Utrecht. Widely known for his work on secretions of the pituitary gland, his work on muscle tension gained such acclaim that he was nominated for the Nobel Prize in 1927. Tragically, his sudden death prevented him from receiving the award. In pharmacology, Magnus is most noted for his pioneering work in the use of isolated tissues. A basic tenet of pharmacological research is that all experimentally derived dependent variables (i.e., potency, drug activity) depend upon an accurate value for drug concentration at the target.

Magnus pioneered an apparatus that could sustain an isolated tissue physiologically for many hours, thereby allowing the measurement of drug effect in a quantitative fashion. The drug was added to a chamber of constant volume ensuring that the concentration of drug acting on the tissue was constant.

(arithmetic and/or statistical) since pEC_{50}s (but not EC_{50}s) are normally distributed. In this example, 50% of the maximal effect is produced by a drug concentration of 10^{-6} M. The negative logarithm of this number is the pEC_{50}, in this case 6.0. The other observed effect is the maximal response. It will be seen that the potency and maximal response of a drug depend on different molecular properties, with the maximal response being primarily dependent on the drug's efficacy (Fig. 1.5B). Figure 1.6A summarizes the characteristics of a semi-logarithmic dose–response curve. In this example, the maximal response is expressed as a fraction (or percentage) of the maximal capability of the system (called the system maximal response). The maximal response to the drug being studied may or may not equal the system maximal response.

It is worth describing some general drug nomenclature at this point; this nomenclature is based on the behavior of a drug in a particular system which may change in different

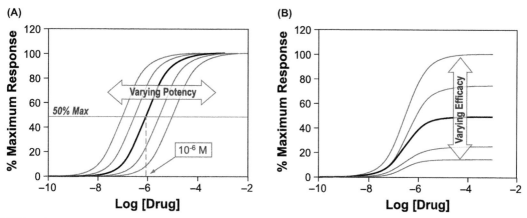

FIGURE 1.5 Two measures of drug activity in a cellular system. (A) The location parameter along the concentration axis represents the drug potency. This is usually quantified by the molar concentration that is seen to produce 50% of the maximal response. For the solid line dose–response curve the concentration producing 50% response is 10^{-6} M; this is reported as the negative logarithm of this value (pEC$_{50}$), in this case the pEC$_{50}$ is 6.0. (B) Another measure of drug activity in a system is the maximal response. While the potency is a complex product of both the affinity and efficacy of the drug, the maximal response is solely dependent upon efficacy.

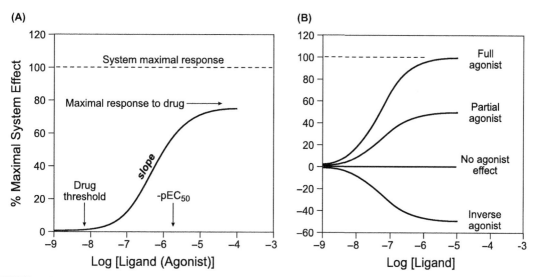

FIGURE 1.6 Features of dose–response curves and different behaviors of drugs characterized by those curves. (A) A dose–response curve is characterized by a threshold effect, a slope of the relationship between dose and response, and a maximal response. This maximal response may or may not equal the maximal response capability of the cell system. (B) The dose–response curve produces a profile of behavior of a drug in a given system. If it produces the maximal response of the system, it is a full agonist; if it produces a sub-maximal response it is a partial agonist. In other cases no observed response may be observed (but the drug may bind to the receptor to be an antagonist). Some systems have an elevated basal response which can then be decreased through drug action; this behavior is inverse agonism.

systems (tissues). In general, a drug that causes a cellular system to change its state and which produces a measurable biological response is referred to as an *agonist*. A drug that produces the maximal response of the system (a maximal response equal to the maximal capability of the system to report cellular response) is termed a *full agonist* (Fig. 1.6B). It should also be noted that a drug may not produce a response equal to the maximal response capability of the system, i.e., a given drug may only produce a maximal response that is below the maximal capability of the system. When this occurs, the drug is referred to as a *partial agonist*. A drug that reduces the biological effect of another drug is called an *antagonist*. An antagonist may itself produce a low level of direct response (i.e., a partial agonist can produce antagonism of responses to full agonists). Finally, there are cases where the tissue itself possesses an elevated basal activity due to a spontaneous activation of receptors. A class of drug that reverses such elevated basal effect is termed an *inverse agonist*; these will be described in later discussions of antagonists (see Chapter 4). It will be seen that the common currency of pharmacology in describing drug effect is the dose–response curve. As a prerequisite to a discussion of these properties, it is useful to describe the cellular target that responds to agonists to yield observable cellular response, in this case the receptor.

LINKING OBSERVED PHARMACOLOGY WITH MOLECULAR MECHANISM

Drug targets are coupled to the organism (cell, organ) through a myriad of biochemical reactions, and these can vary with different cell types. However, these reactions are similar in terms of how they relate input (the stimulus at the start of the process) to output (the result of

activating the process). Specifically, the reactions that link cell surface signaling to cytosolic response are saturable (they reach a finite endpoint with infinite stimulation); an example of such a process is shown in Fig. 1.7. This figure shows a typical relationship between the input to a biochemical reaction (x-axis, to be referred to as the stimulus) and output (y-axis, to be referred to as the response), i.e., low levels of stimulus cause the most change in output until a maximal output is attained. This is consistent with the idea that, in the absence of stimulus, the system is open to activation; therefore, the first molecules interacting have the most opportunity to produce response. As the level of stimulus increases, the probability that new stimulus will encounter a part of the system already interacting with previous stimulus increases and the new output is reduced. Finally, at very high levels of stimulus, the system is maximally engaged and no further response can be elicited.

In addition to saturability, the curved relationship between stimulus and response leads to amplification. For example, in Fig. 1.7, 20% maximal stimulus leads to 64% maximal response. This type of amplification is compounded when such saturable reactions are in series, as often occurs in cells (Fig. 1.8). The nature, capacity and sensitivity of the biochemical reactions linking stimulus and response vary from cell to cell; in fact, this is one way that a cell can tailor its sensitivity to input to its needs. This will be referred to as the efficiency of coupling. This fact precludes the direct linking of the actual sensitivity of the organ to the effect of the drug on the biochemical process; the target coupling process intervenes in a variable way.

There are two main cell-based control points for cellular sensitivity mediated by a pharmacological target; the number of targets available to produce stimulus and the efficiency of coupling of the target to cellular metabolism. Cells use both of these control points to

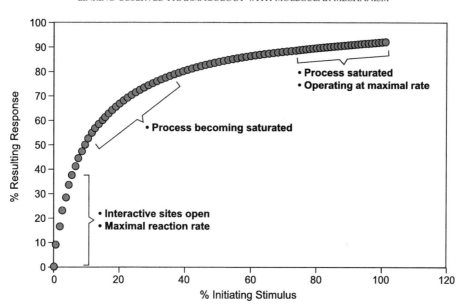

FIGURE 1.7 Depiction of a saturable biochemical process (as would be operative in working cells). The x-axis shows the incoming signal and the y-axis the resulting response. The initial steep rise reflects the fact that the system is open to stimulation; as the system becomes engaged, fewer open sites are present and the slope of the response curve decreases. Once the interacting sites are occupied, no further stimulus can cause increased response, i.e., the response is the maximal response that the process can return.

maintain appropriate levels of stimulus to sustain their function. Differences in target density levels and the components of the cell that control the efficiency of coupling of the target are what cause drugs to have a wide range of potencies and activities in different cell types. It is this variation that must be dealt with and accounted for when drug activity is assessed in a test system for prediction of effect in a therapeutic one.

Agonist effect results from the interplay of four factors; two are related to the drug and two to the system. The drug effects are:

- **Affinity**: The force(s) that cause the agonist and the protein target to interact with each other, i.e., what causes the drug to bind to the target.
- **Efficacy**: The property of the drug that causes the target to change its behavior toward the host cell once the drug is bound.

These drug-related properties are what can be quantified in pharmacological procedures to characterize drug activity. The result of the interaction of the drug with the target provides the cell with a stimulus, i.e., each target furnishes a degree of stimulus to the cell commensurate with the drug's target occupancy (controlled by the concentration of drug and its affinity for the target) and efficacy. Two cell-based properties control the overall stimulus received by the cell. These are:

- **Target density**: The actual number of responding target units exposed to the drug, i.e., receptors on the cell surface.
- **Target coupling efficiency**: The efficiency with which each target is coupled to the cellular response machinery. The series of biochemical processes linking target activation with final cellular response is referred to as stimulus–response coupling.

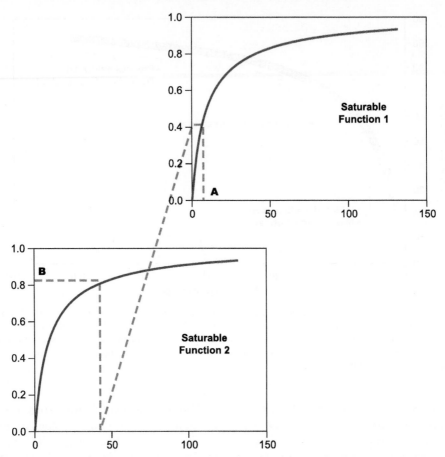

FIGURE 1.8   Amplification of cell signaling through a series arrangement of saturable functions. A stimulus level point A (10%) enters the first saturable function 1 to return a response 1 of 40%. This response then becomes the stimulus input to a second saturable function 2 to yield a further amplified response 2 of 83% (point B). In general, such series signaling can produce very large amplification of minute signals in cells.

Each process along the stimulus−response chain, beginning with the binding of the drug to the target, can be described with a dose−response curve. As seen in Fig. 1.8, as successive biochemical reactions feed into each other (i.e., the response of one reaction becomes the stimulus for the next), amplification occurs. Therefore, the potency of the drug, as the process is viewed further down the stimulus−response chain of reactions, increases. This effect causes the potency for the final effect of the drug to be considerably higher than it is for the first initiating reaction (binding to the target).

The main pharmacological tool used to negate the variable effect of biochemical target-coupling is the null method. Through this device, drugs are compared in terms of their potency (the concentration of drug needed to produce a defined response) to produce a common effect. This imposes the condition that the stimulus of each drug to the cell is subject to

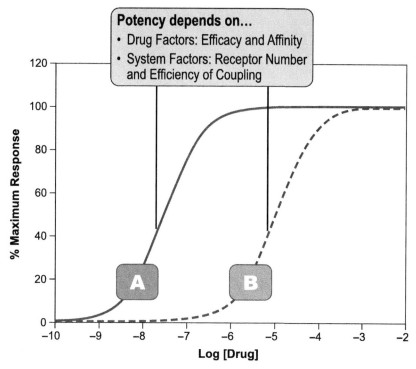

FIGURE 1.9   Dose–response curves to two agonists (A and B). Their respective potencies depend upon the two drug factors of affinity and efficacy, and two tissue factors of receptor number and efficiency of receptor coupling. The null method compares equal responses (for example, the concentrations of each agonist producing 50% of maximal response); this ratio is still dependent upon the drug factors (the respective affinities and efficacies of the agonists), but the tissue factors are common to both and thus cancel each other. This potency ratio is a system-independent measure of the relative affinity and efficacy of the two agonists.

the *same system-dependent modification* and therefore, this effect will cancel when two drugs are compared in the same system (see Fig. 1.9). Through the use of null methods, the relative potency of agonists can be compared in one system to yield a parameter (relative potency ratio) that may be constant for all systems. There is a major assumption required for this method, and this is that the agonists involved activate the target receptor in the same manner, i.e., produce the same receptor active state. There are cases where this is true and other cases where it is *not*. In the cases where it is not true, the relative potency of agonists in whole cell systems is not constant and

thus cannot be used for therapeutic predictions. Chapter 3 discusses these various cases in more detail.

DESCRIPTIVE PHARMACOLOGY: I

This monograph is designed to guide the reader in the application of pharmacological principles to describe the biological activity of drugs. At the end of each chapter, the specific progress towards this end will be summarized. As shown in Fig. 1.10, a new chemical entity (which may or may not be a drug) is tested in a biological preparation and one of two

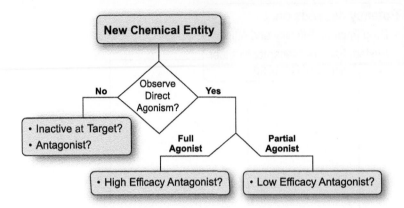

FIGURE 1.10 Schematic diagram of logical progression for determination of drug effect. The end result of this progression at this point is to determine if the new chemical entity produces a visible effect in a pharmacologic assay and, if so, to describe some characteristics of that effect, namely a statement describing efficacy (full or partial agonism) and potency. It should be stressed that this analysis is necessarily linked to the particular assay used to make the measurements, and also that a specific target-based effect requires separate testing of selectivity before conclusions can link effect with specific target activation.

outcomes may result. The chemical may not produce a visible response and this may be due to the fact that it does not bind to and activate the target (inactive), or it does bind but has such a low efficacy that no change in the state of the cell can be observed. The presence of the chemical on the target may preclude further activation of the target by other molecules in which case the chemical is an antagonist; a further set of tests can then be done to define this activity (see Chapters 4 and 5). If an agonist response is observed in the preparation, then this suggests that the chemical has efficacy and may be an agonist. It should be stressed that specific tests for selectivity must be carried out before this conclusion is firm; these are described in Chapter 3. The assay may also show the chemical to be a full or partial agonist; this is a general measure of the strength of efficacy of the test substance. This also underscores a general tenet for a complete analysis at this stage of testing, namely that the classifications of the new chemical entity will still be uniquely tied to the particular biological preparation in which the testing is done. It will be seen in subsequent chapters that a different assay may show what previously appeared to be an antagonist to be an

agonist, and *vice versa*. Also, many low efficacy agonists can produce partial agonism in some tissues and full agonism in others. For this reason, observations made in a single test system must be considered to be system-dependent and subject to change when tests are conducted in other tissues. Procedures outlined in the next chapters will extend these approaches to obtain measures of drug activity that are independent of the test system and thus can be used to predict drug activity in all systems.

At this stage, tests done in a given system (or person) can yield general statements such as:

- The compound produces no observed effect in the system.
- The compound produces partial or full agonism with a potency of x mg/kg (if tests done *in vivo*) or a pEC_{50} of x (if tests done *in vitro*).

SUMMARY

- Drugs bind to and activate biochemical targets in physiological systems.
- Identification of these targets enables chemical access to modify physiology.

- Drugs that produce observed change in cellular processes are termed agonists; those that block such effects are antagonists.
- Agonist effect can concisely be described with a dose−response curve which relates drug effect to drug concentration. The properties of potency and maximal response describe the effect of the agonist in any given system.
- Cells amplify initial chemical signals through a series of saturable biochemical processes; this produces a difference in the dose−response curves describing the initial interaction of the agonist with the receptor and the dose−response curve for cellular response.
- The observed potency of an agonist depends upon two drug-related parameters (affinity, efficacy) and two cell-dependent parameters (target density and efficiency of target coupling).
- The cell-dependent factors can be cancelled when the relative potency of agonists is compared in the same system (null method). Under these circumstances, the observed relative potency reflects differences only in the drug-related parameters of affinity and efficacy (and thus is system-independent). This is true only for agonists that activate the receptor in the same manner.

QUESTIONS

1.1 What is the main value of the receptor concept in pharmacology and physiology?

1.2 How is potency characterized in a dose−response curve?

1.3 Define full agonist, partial agonist, antagonist, inverse agonist.

1.4 Why can the potency of an agonist change when it is tested in different tissues?

1.5 Upon what major assumption is the null method for comparing agonist potency based?

References

[1] A.L. Hopkins, C.R. Groom, The druggable genome, Nature Rev. Drug Disc. 1 (2002) 727−730.

[2] A.D. Luster, Mechanisms of disease: Chemokines − chemotactic cytokines that mediate inflammation, N. Eng. J. Med. 338 (1998) 436−445.

[3] M. Zaitseva, A. Blauvelt, S. Lee, C.K. Lapham, V. Klaus-Kovtun, H. Mostowski, et al., Expression and function of CCR5 and CXCR4 on human langerhans cells and macrophages: Implications for HIV primary infection, Nat. Med. 3 (1997) 1369−1375.

[4] L. Cagnon, J.J. Rossi, Downregulation of the CCR5 beta-chemokine receptor and inhibition of HIV-1 infection by stable VA1-ribozyme chimeric transcripts, Antisense Nucleic Acid Drug Dev. 10 (2000) 251−261.

[5] M.P. Martin, M. Dean, M.W. Smith, C. Winkler, B. Gerrard, N.L. Michael, et al., Genetic acceleration of AIDS progression by promoter variant of CCR5, Science 282 (1998) 1907−1911.

[6] D.N. Cook, M.A. Beck, T.M. Coffman, S.L. Kirby, J.F. Sheridan, I.B. Pragnell, et al., Requirement of MIP-1α for an inflammatory response to viral infection, Science 269 (1995) 1583−1585.

[7] M. Baba, O. Nishimura, N. Kanzaki, M. Okamoto, H. Sawada, Y. Iizawa, et al., A small-molecule, nonpeptide CCR5 antagonist with highly potent and selective anti-HIV-1 activity, Proc. Natl. Acad. Sci. USA 96 (1999) 5698−5703.

[8] F. Cocchi, A.L. De Vico, A. Garzino-Demo, S.K. Arya, R.C. Gallo, P. Lusso, Identification of RANTES, MIP-1, and MIP-1 as the major HIV-suppressive factors produced by CD8 + T cells, Science 270 (1995) 1811−1815.

[9] P.E. Finke, B. Oates, S.G. Mills, M. MacCoss, L. Malkowitz, M.S. Springer, et al., Antagonists of the human CCR5 receptor as anti-HIV-1 agents. Part 4: Synthesis and structure − Activity relationships for 1-[N-(Methyl)-N-(phenylsulfonyl)amino]-2-(phenyl)-4-(4-(N-(alkyl)-N-(benzyloxycarbonyl)amino)piperidin-1-yl)butanes, Bioorg. Med. Chem. Lett. 11 (2001) 2475−2479.

[10] M. Mack, B. Luckow, P.J. Nelson, J. Cihak, G. Simmons, P.R. Clapham, et al., Aminooxypentane-RANTES induces CCR5 internalization but inhibits recycling: A novel inhibitory mechanism of HIV infectivity, J. Exp. Med. 187 (1998) 1215−1224.

[11] G. Simmons, P.R. Clapham, L. Picard, R.E. Offord, M.M. Rosenkilde, T.W. Schwartz, et al., Potent inhibition of HIV-1 infectivity in macrophages and lymphocytes by a novel CCR5 antagonist, Science 276 (1997) 276−279.

[12] A. Garzino-Demo, R.B. Moss, J.B. Margolick, F. Cleghorn, A. Sill, W.A. Blattner, et al., Spontaneous and antigen-induced production of HIV-inhibitory-chemokines is associated with AIDS-free status, Proc. Natl. Acad. Sci. USA 96 (1999) 11986–11991.

[13] H. Ullum, A.C. Lepri, J. Victor, H. Aladdin, A.N. Phillips, J. Gerstoft, et al., Production of beta-chemokines in human immunodeficiency virus (HIV) infection: Evidence that high levels of macrophage in inflammatory protein-1-beta are associated with a decreased risk of HIV progression, J. Infect. Dis. 177 (1998) 331–336.

[14] M. Dean, M. Carrington, C. Winkler, G.A. Huttley, M.W. Smith, R. Allikmets, et al., Genetic restriction of HIV-1 infection and progression to AIDS by a deletion allele of the CKR5 structural gene, Science 273 (1996) 1856–1862.

[15] Y. Huang, W.A. Paxton, S.M. Wolinsky, A.U. Neumann, L. Zhang, T. He, et al., The role of a mutant CCR5 allele in HIV-1 transmission and disease progression, Nat. Med. 2 (1996) 1240–1243.

[16] R. Liu, W.A. Paxton, S. Choe, D. Ceradini, S.R. Martin, R. Horuk, et al., Homozygous defect in HIV-1 coreceptor accounts for resistance of some multiply-exposed individuals to HIV-1 infection, Cell 86 (1996) 367–377.

[17] W.A. Paxton, S.R. Martin, D. Tse, T.R. O'Brien, J. Skurnick, N.L. VanDevanter, et al., Relative resistance to HIV-1 infection of CD4 lymphocytes from persons who remain uninfected despite multiple high-risk sexual exposures, Nat. Med. 2 (1996) 412–417.

[18] M. Samson, F. Libert, B.J. Doranz, J. Rucker, C. Liesnard, C.M. Farber, et al., Resistance to HIV-1 infection in Caucasian individuals bearing mutant alleles to the CCR-5 chemokine recepetor gene, Nature 382 (1996) 722–725.

2

Drug Affinity and Efficacy

By the end of this chapter the reader should understand the concept of a molecule having an "affinity" for a protein, and what the uniquely pharmacologic concept of "efficacy" means and its mechanism. The reader should also understand how drugs can have many efficacies, and how these can be expressed in either "full" or "partial" agonism. The reader will also see how particular methods to compare full and partial agonists with respect to relative activity are used in discovery.

INTRODUCTION

Up to this point, drug activity (specifically that of an agonist) is described as observed effect quantified by a dose—response curve. Thus the maximal response and the potency of an agonist (location of the curve along the

drug concentration axis) in any specific system yield the measure of activity in that system. Also, as noted in the last chapter, the magnitude of the observed organ response is controlled by four factors, two drug-related and two tissue-related. This chapter describes the two drug related parameters of *affinity* and *efficacy*. The value in quantifying these parameters is that they are unique properties of the drug acting on the target, and thus are true for that target in all tissues and organs in which it resides. Therefore, if the affinity and efficacy of a given molecule can be determined in one system (referred to as the "test" system), then these parameters may be used to assess drug activity in any other system, including the therapeutic one. This is of great value since drugs are very rarely discovered and studied directly in the therapeutic system. A prerequisite to the determination of the affinity and efficacy of agonists is to know that the agonism is selective for the particular target of interest. There are two main strategies for making this determination.

NEW TERMINOLOGY

- k_1: The rate of association of a molecule as it binds to the target in units of $s^{-1} mol^{-1}$.
- k_2: The rate of dissociation of the molecule away from the target during the binding process in units of s^{-1}.
- K_{eq}: Equilibrium dissociation constant of the molecule–target complex in units of mole ($K_{eq} = k_2/k_1$); also equal to the concentration of drug that binds to 50% of the target population available for binding. For agonists, K_{eq} is denoted K_A; for antagonists K_B. Affinity = K_{eq}^{-1}.
- **Lead**: In new drug discovery, a molecule that fulfills criteria for possible activity from a screening process is termed a "hit." A hit with the added qualities of chemical tractability (opportunity to change the chemical scaffold to modify structure), selectivity and lack of toxicity is termed a "lead."
- **Lead optimization**: The process of iterative medicinal chemistry to modify structure to enhance primary activity and selectivity.

AGONIST SELECTIVITY

As discussed in the previous chapter, there are numerous potential biological targets in any given cell that a chemical could activate to cause agonism. Usually, a non-specific activation is not therapeutically useful, as it comes with a non-specific activation of organs leading to unwanted side-effects. By definition, the chemical control of pathology through pharmacological agonism requires a selective activation of the predetermined therapeutic

biological target. There are two basic approaches for identifying selective agonist effect.

The first is pharmacologic intervention whereby a specific antagonist of the target is given as a pretreatment to the preparation (either *in vitro* or *in vivo*) to see if the observed agonism to the test agonist is eliminated (or ablated) (see Fig. 2.1). If the agonist action emanates from the binding of the test agonist to the same site as that utilized by the antagonist, a steric hindrance will occur and agonism will be blocked. However, it will be seen that in the case of an allosteric activation of the target where the test agonist binds to a site separate from that of the antagonist, interference of the agonist response with antagonist binding may not occur. Therefore, another strategy that may be employed in these cases (or in general to ensure that this possibility is considered experimentally) is to use a recombinant system. In this approach, genetic material for the biological target of interest (specifically complementary DNA (cDNA)) is used to transfect host cells. The test agonist is then tested in the transfected cell and the non-transfected host cell (i.e., the same cell line but with no receptor present). If the response is observed only in the transfected cell line (containing the target of interest), this is presumptive evidence that the agonist activates the biological target of interest (see Fig. 2.1).

AFFINITY

A simple model of ligand binding, originally designed to describe the binding of chemicals to metal surfaces in the making of filaments for light bulbs, was published by the chemist Irving Langmuir (see Box 2.1); accordingly, it is referred to as the Langmuir adsorption isotherm and it still forms the basis for the measurement and quantification of drug affinity. In Langmuir's model, a drug molecule has an intrinsic **rate of association** with the

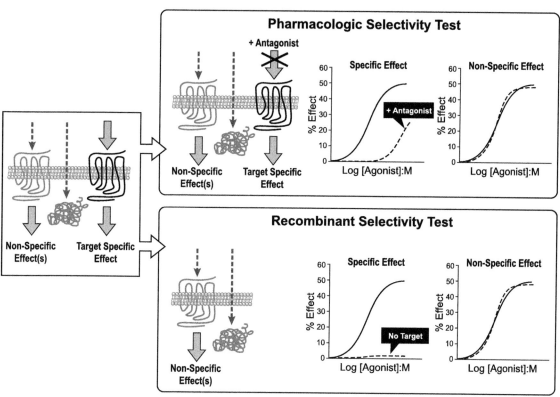

FIGURE 2.1 Two methods to determine the specificity of agonism. A given agonist may activate a specific biological target (solid arrows) or cause response through activation of elements within the cellular host (dashed arrows). Specific target activation can be confirmed by specific blockade of the response with a specific antagonist for the target ("Pharmacologic Selectivity Test"). Alternatively, if recombinant cells consisting of host cells containing and not containing the target are available, the observance of a response to the agonist only in cells containing the target provides presumptive evidence of selective agonism ("Recombinant Selectivity Test").

receptor (referred to as the "rate of condensation" by Langmuir). In Langmuir's system the target was the surface of metal, but in the context of pharmacology the target is the binding pocket of a biologically relevant protein such as a receptor. This rate of association (denoted k_1) is driven by changes in energy, i.e., the energy of the system containing the drug in the receptor binding pocket is lower than the energy of the system with the drug not bound in the pocket. The drug also has a *rate of dissociation* from the receptor (referred to by Langmuir as a rate of "evaporation") which

describes the change in energy when the molecule diffuses away from the surface (denoted k_2). When a drug is present in the compartment containing the receptor, then the concentration gradient controls the movement of drug molecules. The absence of drug in the receptor binding pocket drives the binding reaction toward drug binding to the receptor but, as more drug binds, the bound drug will diffuse out of the binding pocket in accordance with its natural tendency to do so. This leads to an equilibrium whereby the rate of drug leaving the binding pocket will equal the rate

BOX 2.1

IRVING LANGMUIR AND THE LANGMUIR ADSORPTION ISOTHERM

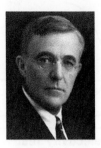

Irving Langmuir 1881–1957

Irving Langmuir (born in Brooklyn, New York) graduated as a metallurgical engineer from the School of Mines at Columbia University in 1903. He went on to achieve a

PhD in Physical Chemistry with Nersnt. He returned to America to join, and eventually become director of, the Research Laboratory of the General Electric Company in Schnectady, New York. Langmuir's studies of vacuum phenomena led him to investigate the properties of adsorbed films, leading to his derivation of the adsorption isotherm. He contributed to the Lewis theory of shared electrons and his work led to the gas-filled incandescent lamp and the discovery of atomic hydrogen. Langmuir won numerous awards for his work, including the Nobel Prize for Chemistry in 1932.

of drug approaching and entering the binding pocket. The ratio of k_2/k_1 determines the amount of drug bound to the receptor at any one instant and this becomes a measure of how well the drug binds to the receptor. This ratio is referred to as the equilibrium dissociation constant of the drug–receptor complex (denoted K_{eq}). Under these circumstances, the reciprocal of K_{eq} is a measure of the affinity of the chemical for the target. The derivation of Langmuir's isotherm, in his original terminology, is given in Box 2.2; the form utilized by pharmacologists is:

$$\rho_A = \frac{[A]}{[A] + K_{eq}} \qquad (2.1)$$

When the concentration of the drug is equal to K_{eq}, then $\rho = 0.5$, i.e., the K_{eq} is the concentration of drug that occupies 50% of the available receptor population. Therefore, the magnitude of K_{eq} is inversely proportional to the affinity of the drug for the receptor. For

example, consider two drugs one with $K_{eq} = 10^{-9}$ M and another with $K_{eq} = 10^{-7}$ M. The first drug occupies 50% of the receptors at a concentration 1/100 of that required by the second. Clearly the drug with $K_{eq} = 10^{-9}$ has a higher affinity for the receptor than the one with $K_{eq} = 10^{-7}$ M.

It can be seen from equation 2.1 that, for a ligand with K_{eq} of 10^{-7} M (100 nM), the fraction of sites bound can be calculated for any concentration (for example, 30 nM would occupy (30 nM)/(30 nM + 100 nm) = 23% of the sites. In fact, equation 2.1 enables the calculation of a complete binding curve. Experimentally, if the binding of a series of concentrations can be measured, then a relationship between concentration and percent bound can be determined (Fig. 2.2). As is the case with dose–response curves, these curves are best described using a semi-logarithmic format (see Fig. 2.2). Assuming that a direct measure of the amount of bound ligand can be

BOX 2.2

DERIVATION OF LANGMUIR'S ISOTHERM

Langmuir's model was centered on the calculation of the fraction of the total area of surface bound by a chemical (denoted by Langmuir as θ_μ). The fraction of total area left free for further binding of new molecule to the surface is given by $1 - \theta_\mu$. In Langmuir's terminology, the amount of chemical bound to the surface is the product of the concentration of drug available for binding (denoted as μ), the rate of "condensation" of chemical onto the surface (α) and the fraction of surface left free for further binding $(1 - \theta_\mu)$ (Rate of condensation $= \mu\alpha[1 - \theta_\mu]$). Similarly, the amount of drug diffusing away (denoted "evaporation" by Langmuir) from the surface is given by the amount already bound (θ_μ) multiplied by a rate of evaporation (denoted V_1) (Rate of evaporation $= \theta_\mu V_1$).

At equilibrium, the fractional amount diffusing toward the receptor is equal to the fractional amount diffusing away from the receptor:

$$\mu\alpha[1 - \theta_\mu] = \theta_\mu V_1$$

Rearranging to isolate θ_μ, the fraction of chemical bound to the surface yields:

$$\theta_\mu = \frac{\alpha\mu}{\alpha\mu + V_1}$$

Pharmacologists and biochemists define the fraction of biological target bound by a chemical (denoted A) as ρ_A and α as k_1 (a rate of association with the target), V_1 as k_2 (rate of dissociation from the target) and combine k_1 and k_2 into an equilibrium dissociation constant denoted K_{eq} ($K_{eq} = k_2/k_1$).

$$\rho_A = \frac{[A]}{[A] + K_{eq}}$$

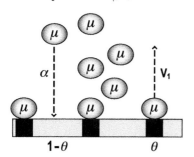

made (for instance, if the ligand is radioactive and the quantity of radioactive–ligand complex could be quantified), then K_{eq} can be measured directly; this can be accomplished with saturation binding experiments with radioactive ligands.

Under certain circumstances, the affinity of an agonist may also be directly observed from agonist effect. Specifically, the EC_{50} value for a *partial agonist* is a good approximation of the affinity for the agonist. The reason for this

effect is the fact that a partial agonist does not saturate the stimulus–response capability of the tissue; therefore the maximal receptor occupancy can be identified through observation of the functional maximal response. Under these circumstances the response to a partial agonist is proportional to the receptor occupancy. Therefore, the EC_{50} of the partial agonist becomes a reasonable approximation of the concentration of agonist occupying 50% of the available receptors; by definition the K_{eq}

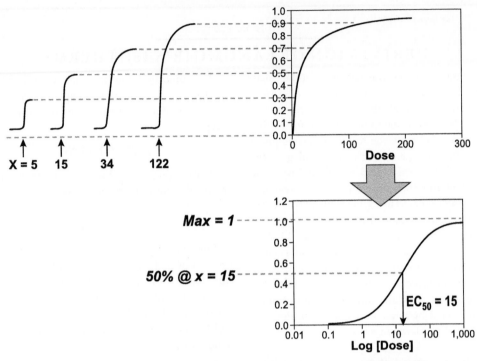

FIGURE 2.2   Binding defined by the Langmuir adsorption isotherm. Different concentrations of ligand, when added to the preparation, bind different fractions of the available binding sites according to a curve defined by the adsorption isotherm. This defines a curved relationship which is sigmoidal when plotted on a semi-logarithmic axis (Log Dose versus fraction of sites bound). The midpoint of this sigmoidal relationship is the EC_{50}, the concentration binding to 50% of the available sites.

for receptor binding (the affinity of a partial agonist $= 1/K_{eq} = 1/EC_{50}$) can directly be obtained from the dose–response curve for a partial agonist) (see Fig. 2.3).

Unfortunately, the same simple relationship does not hold for the EC_{50} of a full agonist and agonist affinity. This is because the maximal response to the full agonist cannot be reliably related to 100% receptor occupancy (in fact, the opposite is true). Due to the amplifying effect of agonist response by cells (specifically agonist efficacy coupled with the cellular effects of high target densities and efficient target-coupling mechanisms to cellular response; see Chapter 1), the receptor binding curve is displaced to the right of the observed agonism. Because of this effect, the EC_{50} of a curve to a full agonist will be lower than the concentration that occupies 50% of the target sites, i.e., it is no longer an estimate for K_{eq} (1/Affinity). In fact, the magnitude of the EC_{50} for a full agonist is a complex function of the affinity and the efficacy of the agonist (see Derivations and Proofs, Appendix B) and also the effect of stimulus–response amplification by the tissue (Fig. 2.4).

Agonist response can be characterized in a system-independent manner by measurement of the affinity and efficacy of the agonist; this will be described in more detail in the following chapter. However, while both the parameters of affinity and efficacy are required to describe agonists, only affinity is required to characterize the activity of target antagonists

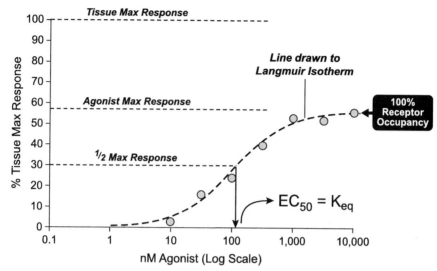

FIGURE 2.3   Dose–response curve for a partial agonist. If the maximal response to the agonist is lower than the system maximal response, then the concentration producing maximal response approximates the saturation binding concentation of the agonist (concentration binding to 100% of the available receptors). Under these circumstances the EC_{50} of the curve also approximates the K_{eq} for binding (concentration binding to 50% of the sites).

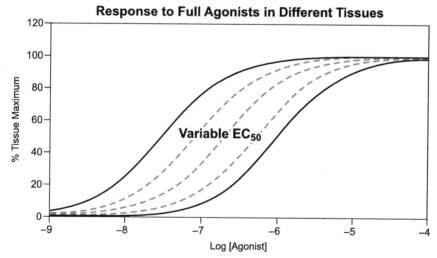

FIGURE 2.4   In contrast to curves for partial agonists (see Fig. 2.3), changes in cellular sensitivity to full agonists result in variation in the EC_{50}. However, the EC_{50} is a complex function of both the affinity and efficacy of the agonist; therefore, no specific information about the affinity of the full agonist can be derived from the EC_{50}.

(molecules that block the activation of the target by agonists). The various methods employed to measure the affinity of antagonists will be described in Chapters 4 and 5.

EFFICACY

The property of a molecule that causes the target to change its behavior toward the cellular host when the molecule is bound to the target is called *efficacy*. However small a drug molecule may be compared to the receptor protein, the receptor with drug bound to it is a different thermodynamic species than the receptor with no drug bound. Therefore, by definition, there is a property imparted to the receptor through the binding of a drug. The term *efficacy* was coined by the Scottish pharmacologist R. P. Stephenson (see Box 2.3). The compelling observation in these studies was the fact that a collection of highly related alkyltrimethylammonium partial agonists produced

contractions of guinea pig ileum with nearly identical affinity (pEC_{50}), but with varying maximal response (see Fig. 2.5).[1] These data made it apparent that there must be another drug-related property causing these molecules to have differing capabilities of inducing response; this property was given the name efficacy. While Stephenson defined efficacy as both a drug-related and a tissue-related property, it will be seen that there are pharmacological procedures that allow the cancellation of the tissue-dependent aspects of efficacy to allow it to be used as a strictly drug-dependent parameter (*vide infra*).

The most common setting for observing efficacy is in the effect of agonists on cellular systems. On a molecular scale, it is useful to consider how an agonist elicits a change in the receptor to cause cellular activation. Whereas enzymes bind their substrates in energetically constrained conformations to stretch bonds to a breaking point (or to create a new bond), receptors do not change their "substrates," nor

---

BOX 2.3

R. P. STEPHENSON AND DRUG "EFFICACY"

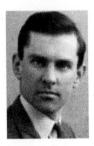

R. P. Stephenson 1925–2004

Robert Stephenson, renowned for introducing the concept of efficacy into pharmacology, was an English pharmacologist who worked in the Pharmacology Department in Edinburgh University. He studied the activity of

alkyltrimethylammonium compounds as contractile agonists in guinea pig ileum through activation of muscarinic receptors. It was here he noted that, while the compounds had fairly uniform affinity for the receptors, they differed considerably in their ability to cause contraction. This led him to postulate that the compounds need to have another intrinsic property to differentiate one from the other; he gave this fundamental property of drugs the name efficacy. Stephenson considered both the intrinsic efficacy of the agonist and the sensitivity of the tissue to be a combined description of the efficacy of an agonist in any tissue.

are they permanently altered by their interaction with drugs. Instead, an agonist activates the receptor when it binds and the activation ceases when the agonist diffuses away. Historically, it was thought that the binding of the drug deformed the receptor and produced an activated state through drug binding (protein conformational induction). However, such a mechanism is energetically extremely unfavorable. In thermodynamic terms, a much more reasonable mechanism is through protein *conformational selection* (see Fig. 2.6). In this scheme, drugs bind to a limited number of pre-existing receptor conformations and stabilize those through binding (at the expense of other conformations – Le Chatelier's principle of an equilibrium responding to perturbation – see Box 2.4). Because of the selective affinity of the ligand for receptor active states a bias in the collection of conformations

results. If two conformations are inter-convertible, then a ligand with higher affinity for one of the conformations will enrich the system with this conformation at the expense of other conformations. The mathematical description of how this occurs is given in Box 2.5. This defines binding as an active, not a passive, process. Specifically, if a ligand has selective affinity for a collection of protein conformations, it will actively change the make-up of that collection. It is this active property of ligands that can result in physiological cellular response (efficacy).

Affinity and efficacy can be dissociable properties that vary independently with changes in chemical structure (i.e., see Fig. 2.5). It is useful to note the independence of affinity and efficacy on chemical structure for drug development, as these properties can be manipulated separately *en route* to a defined therapeutic

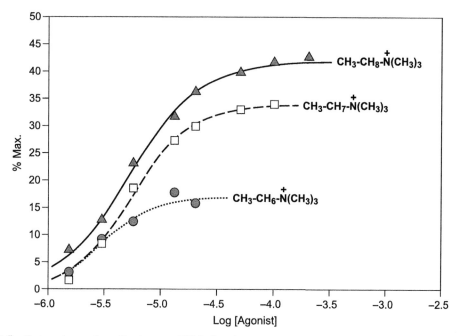

FIGURE 2.5 Data redrawn from Stephenson (1956) showing contractions of guinea pig ileum to three alkyltrimethylammonium partial agonists. While these molecules are of comparable affinity for the muscarinic receptors in this preparation, clearly the molecules differ in their ability to induce maximal response. Stephenson reasoned that the critical property causing these differences is efficacy.

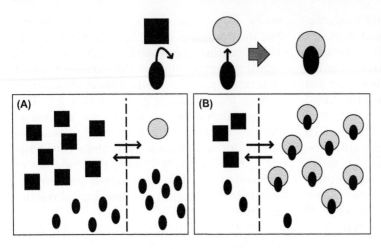

FIGURE 2.6 Conformational Selection as a molecular mechanism for efficacy. The system is comprised of two protein conformations (squares and circles) in equilibrium with each other. A given ligand (dark oval) does not bind well to the inactive state of the receptor (filled squares), but rather selectively binds to the active state (open circles) producing a new thermodynamic species (open circles bound to ligand). This drives the equilibrium toward the free open circle state causing the system to be enriched in this species. If the open circles induce cellular response, then the ligand is an agonist.

BOX 2.4

LE CHATELIER'S PRINCIPLE

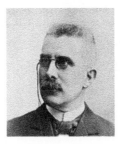

Henry Louis Le Chatelier 1850–1936

Henry Louis Le Chatelier was a French–Italian chemist most famous for devising "Le Chatelier's principle." This idea is used by chemists to predict the effect a change in conditions has on a chemical equilibrium. Although he trained as an engineer, Le Chatelier chose chemistry as a career that went on to explore general chemical laws and principles ("... all my life I maintained a respect for order ... order is one of the most perfect forms..."). His famous principle stated "... If a dynamic equilibrium is disturbed by changing the conditions, the position of equilibrium moves to counteract the change." This concept was first presented to the Academie des Sciences in Paris in 1885. This principle applies to isoenergetic interconvertible protein conformations, and dictates how ligands bias protein ensembles toward active states to produce a cellular response.

---

entity (as in the case of the discovery and synthesis of the important class of histamine receptor H2 antagonists for the treatment of peptic ulcer). In this instance, a chemical effort to enhance the affinity and eliminate the efficacy of the natural agonist histamine for the target H2 receptor resulted in the synthesis of cimetidine, a potent molecule with high affinity for the H2 receptor but no efficacy (see Box 2.6). This molecule competes with histamine to antagonize the production of stomach acid and thus promotes healing of ulcers.

BOX 2.5

PROTEIN CONFORMATIONAL SELECTION

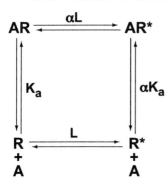

Assume two protein conformations R and R* are controlled by an equilibrium dissociation constant L, where $L = [R^*]/[R]$. Similarly consider a ligand A with an affinity (defined as the equilibrium association constant $K_a = k_1/k_2$) of K_a for receptor state R and αK_a for receptor state R*, where the factor α denotes the differential affinity of the agonist for R*, i.e., $\alpha = 10$ denotes a 10-fold greater affinity of the ligand for the R* state. The effect of α (selective affinity) on the ability of the ligand to alter the equilibrium between R and R* can be calculated by examining the amount of R* (both as R* and AR*) present in the system in the absence of A, and in the presence of A. The equilibrium expression for $([R^*] + [AR^*])/[R_t]$ where $[R_t]$ is the total receptor concentration given by the conservation equation $[R_t] = [R] + [AR] + [R^*] + [AR^*])$ is:

$$\rho = \frac{L(1 + \alpha[A]/K_A)}{[A]/K_A(1 + \alpha L) + L + 1}$$

where K_A is the equilibrium dissociation constant of the agonist–receptor complex. In the absence of agonist ($[A] = 0$), $\rho_0 = L/(1 + L)$, while in the presence of a maximal concentration of ligand (saturating the receptors; $[A] \to \infty$) $\rho_\infty = (\alpha[1 + L])/(1 + \alpha L)$. Therefore, the effect of the ligand on the proportion of the R* state is given by the ratio ρ_∞/ρ_0. This ratio is given by:

$$\frac{\rho_\infty}{\rho_0} = \frac{\alpha(1 + L)}{(1 + \alpha L)}$$

It can be seen from this equation that if the ligand has an equal affinity for both the R and R* states ($\alpha = 1$) then ρ_∞/ρ_0 will equal unity and no change in the proportion of R* will result from maximal ligand binding. However, if $\alpha > 1$, then the presence of the conformationally selective ligand will cause the ratio ρ_∞/ρ_0 to be > 1 and the R* state will be enriched by presence of the ligand. If the R* state promotes physiological response, then ligand A will promote response and be an agonist. This defines binding as an active, not a passive, process. Specifically, if a ligand has selective affinity for a collection of protein conformations, it will actively change the make-up of that collection. It is this active property of ligands that can result in physiological cellular response (efficacy).

DRUGS WITH MULTIPLE EFFICACIES

Up to this point, efficacy has been discussed as if it is a single drug property. In early

considerations of efficacy, test systems were simple and consisted of a single index of tissue response (for example, Stephenson used the *in vitro* contraction of guinea pig ileum). The assumption at that time was that efficacy

BOX 2.6

JAMES BLACK AND DISSOCIATION OF AFFINITY AND EFFICACY

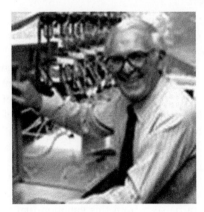

Sir James Black (1924–2010) was a Scottish pharmacologist who discovered two major classes of therapeutic drugs; beta-blockers and H2 histamine antagonists. The discovery of this latter class was based on the principle that the structure activity relationships governing drug affinity and efficacy could be different. His aim was to cure stomach ulcer by blocking the histamine-induced release of acid that prevented ulcers from healing. As stated by Black: "...we knew that the receptor bound histamine, so it was a matter of keeping affinity and losing efficacy..." For his groundbreaking discoveries Black received the Nobel Prize for Medicine in 1988. Below are shown the key molecules that illustrate how efficacy can be reduced and affinity enhanced.

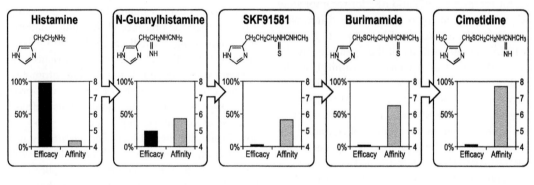

was linear, meaning that it was a reflection of all the biological actions mediated by that target in the cell. Also at that time, receptors were thought to be more simple units controlling single functions (i.e., calcium entry into the cell to mediate contraction). With increasing technology, different assays have been developed that can monitor the functions of receptors and cells, and with this has come an appreciation of how receptors perform multiple tasks and have complex behaviors. Figure 2.7 shows some prominent behaviors of seven transmembrane (7TM) receptors that have been elucidated through separate assay technologies. These proteins can process numerous signals from extracellular molecules to activate different cytosolic signaling proteins, such as G proteins and β-arrestin; these targets also have a dynamic lifetime on the cell surface as they are expressed, reside in the cell

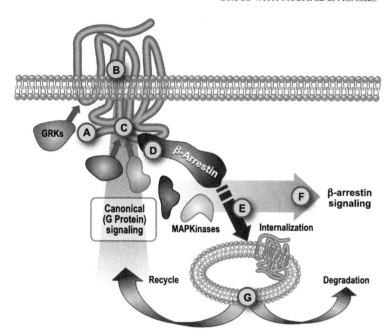

FIGURE 2.7 Seven transmembrane receptors have complex behaviors in cells and these may be exploited therapeutically. Thus, binding of ligands to these proteins can cause activation of signaling proteins called G proteins (C) and subsequent phosphorylation of receptors by G protein receptor kinases (A). These targets may also accommodate binding of allosteric ligands (B — see Chapter 5). These targets also bind the cytosolic molecule β-arrestin (D) which can cause recycling of the receptor to the cell surface or internalization of the receptor into endosomes. Internalized receptor can be degraded (G) or form a scaffold for cytosolic MAPKinases to produce cellular signals (F).

membrane and then disappear into the cytosol again to be recycled or destroyed. Activation of these targets by agonists changes the dynamics of receptor behavior through processes such as phosphorylation by kinases, desensitization and internalization (Fig. 2.7). It is important to realize that different agonists can produce these effects differentially, i.e., not all agonists produce a uniform set of behaviors in 7TM receptors. This being the case, it will be seen that different molecules can have more than one efficacy as they cause activation of different aspects of target behavior. For example, there are agonists that primarily activate only G proteins through a receptor, while other agonists activate only β-arrestin through the same receptor. The mechanism by which this occurs is the formation of different active states of the receptor. For example, Fig. 2.8 shows two agonists designated A and B both activating the same receptor target but selecting different active receptor states that go on to activate different cytosolic coupling proteins (designated C_1 and C_2). There are two major consequences of this mechanism. First, formation of drug-specific receptor active states allows the reduction in the breadth of effect to an agonist with a resulting potential for greater selectivity. Second, this functional selectivity produces varying agonist potencies in whole cells, thereby negating characterizations of potency ratios as system-independent measures of affinity and efficacy of agonists (as was shown in Chapter 1, Fig. 1.9). This is because the actual microscopic efficacy of functionally selective agonists is different. In the case shown in Fig. 2.8, the cellular "efficacy" of agonists A and B may lead to the same general change in cellular state, but the means by which this is achieved on the molecular level differs. Therefore, the relative activities of these agonists depend on the dominance of various cell types for each of the separate signaling pathways. For example, a primarily β-arrestin signaling molecule will be differentially more active in cells containing large amounts of β-arrestin than in cells that do not.

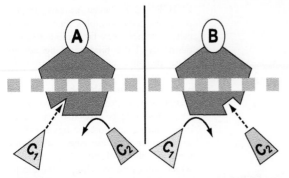

FIGURE 2.8 Functional selectivity of agonist signaling. Agonists A and B may stabilize different active state conformations of the protein to activate different coupling proteins (C_1 and C_2) in the cell. If this occurs, then the cellular relative potency ratios of such agonists in different cells may not be constant.

This can lead to ambiguity in classifying drugs for therapeutic purpose. Specifically, molecules with numerous efficacies can be both agonists for some cellular functions and antagonists for others. For instance, some β-blocker antagonists (antagonists of β-adrenoceptors; see Chapter 4) are also activators (agonists) of Extracellular Receptor Kinases (ERK). Similarly, two agonists could have similar primary activities but different and important secondary properties. For example, while natural hormones and neurotransmitters, such as serotonin (5-HT), produce activation of receptors leading to desensitization and receptor internalization into the cytosol with prolonged activation, there are agonists that produce activation with considerably less desensitization. This type of functional selectivity can lead to superior therapeutic agonism (i.e., sustained opioid analgesia with no tolerance). Another form of functional selectivity defines antagonists that produce no activation but nevertheless produce receptor internalization. Such drugs produce better antagonism in cases where all effect needs to be abolished (internalization of CCR5 receptors for removal of HIV-1 sites of infectious binding).

QUANTIFYING AGONIST ACTIVITY

Under ideal circumstances the affinity and relative efficacy of agonists can be quantified and used in a system-independent manner to predict therapeutic agonism (see Chapter 3). However, even when this is not the case, agonism still can be quantified to describe agonists. The methods for doing this are different for full versus partial agonists. For full agonists, equiactive potency ratios are used. Thus, the ratios of EC_{50} values are used to quantify the relative potency of full agonists. If the agonists produce response by an identical mechanism of activation of the target (i.e., stabilize the same active state of the protein), then these potency ratios are system-independent measures of relative agonist activity. For example, for two agonists of identical mechanism, one with a pEC_{50} of 8.2 and another with a pEC_{50} of 7.1, the potency ratio is $10^{(8.2-7.1)} = 12.6$. This ratio should be true of these two agonists in every tissue where they function as full agonists. An example of ranking full agonists through potency ratios is shown in Fig. 2.9.

More detailed information can be obtained for partial agonists. When the agonist does not produce the system maximal response, as discussed previously, the EC_{50} becomes a surrogate estimate of the K_{eq} for binding to the target (affinity = $1/K_{eq}$). Similarly, the maximal response, although not numerically equal to the efficacy of the agonist, can be used to rank agonists according to a scale of efficacy. Thus, it can be assumed that if the maximal response to a given partial agonist [A] is greater than the maximal response of another partial agonist [B], the efficacy of A is greater than the efficacy of B. An example of how agonist affinity and efficacy can be estimated for partial agonists is shown in Fig. 2.10. In this figure it can be seen that there are different orders of potency for efficacy (maximal response) and affinity (potency); this is a clear indication that

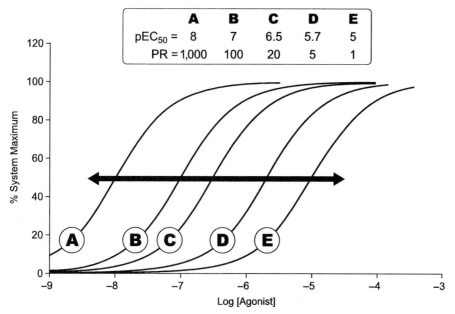

FIGURE 2.9 Quantifying full agonist effect through the measurement of potency ratios. Full agonists A–E have the potencies shown (pEC$_{50}$ values). The relative potencies (measured as the ratio of EC$_{50}$ values) should be constant for these agonists in all cell types if they produce a response through identical mechanisms.

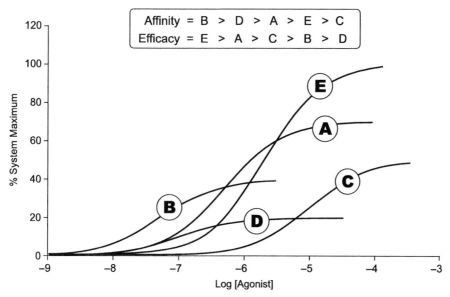

FIGURE 2.10 Characteristics of partial agonist dose–response curves. The EC$_{50}$ values of the curves to partial agonists reflect affinity thus, for the partial agonists shown, the affinities of molecules are B = 30 nM, D = 100 nM, A = 300 nM, E = 1 μM and C ≑ 100 μM. The rank order of efficacy of the agonists can be discerned from the relative maximal responses as shown.

the structural differences in the molecules have different effects on efficacy and affinity.

The behavior of full and partial agonists in cell systems suggests ideal test systems for lead optimization and screening for new drugs. In terms of screening, the most sensitive system possible is best since this will detect weak agonists. In view of the known amplification of signals as they are measured distal to the initial point of initiation (see Derivations and Proofs, Appendix B), the end organ cellular response is optimal for new drug screening. Once a chemical scaffold is identified and medicinal chemists begin to optimize activity, a system where the effect of changing chemical structure on affinity and, separately, on efficacy, is optimal, since much more information can be obtained. As noted in Fig. 2.10, this would be assays in which the agonists demonstrate partial agonist activity.

DESCRIPTIVE PHARMACOLOGY: II

Continuing the process of pharmacologic characterization of new molecules (from

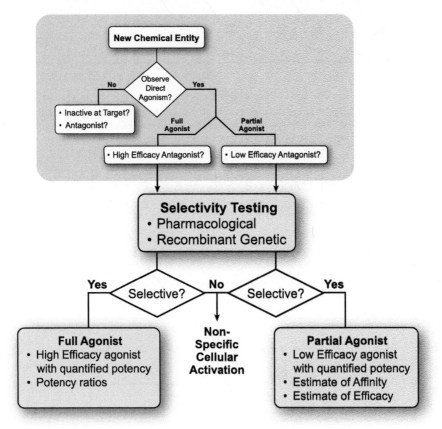

FIGURE 2.11   Continuation of logical progression for determination of new drug effect (from Fig. 1.10). Once agonism has been observed, it must be determined that it is selective for the biological target of interest. If the response is full agonism, then system-independent characterization of relative efficacy (that may transcend cell type) can be made through relative potency ratios (if the agonists produce a response in an identical manner). For partial agonists, the EC_{50} value is an estimate of affinity and the maximal response denotes relative efficacy.

Linking Observed Pharmacology with Molecular Mechanism, Chapter 1), this chapter discusses the characterization of agonists from the point where a cellular response to the molecule has been observed (see Fig. 2.11). The next step is to confirm that the agonism is specifically related to the biological target of interest. It is also possible to begin to characterize the agonism in more detail, either through quantifying full agonist potency ratios or, for partial agonists, estimation of agonist affinity through measurement of the pEC_{50}. Partial agonism also enables the ranking of efficacy through comparison of maximal responses.

SUMMARY

- Specific agonism can be confirmed by determining that specific antagonists of the target block response to the agonist and/or that the presence of the target is required to demonstrate response to the agonist.
- Affinity is quantified through a ratio of the rate of dissociation of the molecule from the protein (k_2) and the rate of association to the protein (k_1) in a parameter referred to as K_{eq} (where $K_{eq} = k_2/k_1$). This is the concentration of ligand that binds to 50% of the available receptors.
- Efficacy is the property of a molecule that changes the behavior of the biological target towards its cellular host when it is bound to that target.
- Molecules can have multiple efficacies depending on which behavior of the biological target is considered.
- Potency ratios can furnish system-independent (constant for all tissues)

measures of relative agonism (providing the agonists have identical modes of action).
- The pEC_{50} value for agonism is a reasonable approximation of the affinity of a partial agonist.
- The maximal response of partial agonists can be used to rank order the efficacy of the partial agonists.
- The ideal assay for new drug screening is a highly sensitive one (end organ response) whereas a good assay for lead optimization is where the agonists produce partial agonism.

QUESTIONS

2.1 The response to a test agonist is not blocked by conventional antagonists of the target. What could be happening?

2.2 Drug A has an equilibrium dissociation constant (K_{eq}) of 10^{-8} M while drug B has a K_{eq} of 10^{-10} M. Which drug has the higher affinity and why?

2.3 Two agonists produce responses in a system both with a pEC_{50} of 7.5. However, one produces 25% maximal response while the other produces 90% maximal response. What is the difference between these two agonists?

2.4 The potency ratio for two full agonists A and B is 15.4 in one cellular system and 2.3 in another. What does this lack of correlation of full agonist potency ratio suggest?

Reference

[1] R.P. Stephenson, A modification of receptor theory, Br. J. Pharmacol. 11 (1956) 379–393.

3

Predicting Agonist Effect

By the end of this chapter readers should be able to use the Black–Leff operational model to quantify agonist affinity and efficacy. They should also be able to use ratios of these values obtained in a test system to predict agonism for the same agonists in any other system.

AGONIST RESPONSE IN DIFFERENT TISSUES

As discussed in Chapter 1, the potency of an agonist depends on the drug-related properties of *affinity* and *efficacy*, and the cell-related properties of target density (number of responding units in the cell) and the efficiency with which these target units are coupled to the cell response producing machinery. These two latter factors vary with cell type, leading to variable potency of any given agonist in different cell types. It is useful to consider the pattern that the dose–response curves to a given agonist will assume in a range of tissues of varying target density and/or target coupling efficiency. As discussed in Chapter 2, the EC_{50} of the curve to a partial agonist is an approximate estimate of the binding K_{eq} (affinity^{-1}). This is a molecular property of the agonist that is constant for all tissues, so it follows that in tissues where the agonist produces partial maximal effect, the EC_{50} will be relatively constant and equal to a value near the K_{eq}. Also as noted in Chapter 2, in more sensitive tissues where full agonism is produced, the EC_{50} dissociates from K_{eq} and becomes a complex function of both affinity and efficacy (see Derivations and Proofs, Appendix B2). With increasing sensitivity of the tissue, the dose–response curve to the full

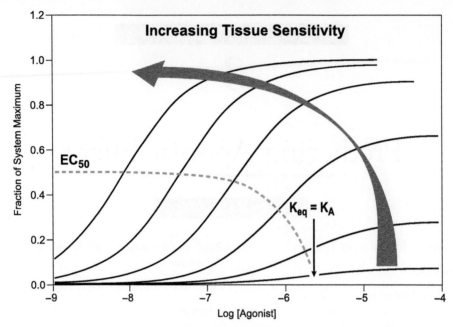

FIGURE 3.1   The effects of increasing tissue sensitivity on response to an agonist. In low sensitivity systems, the curve shows a maximum that is below the tissue maximal response and the EC_{50} can be approximated by the K_{eq} for agonist binding to the receptor (denoted as K_A). As tissue sensitivity increases, the maximal response increases until the tissue maximum is attained. Increases in sensitivity beyond this point have no further effect on the maximal response to the agonist (i.e., the agonist produces the tissue maximum), but do shift the dose–response curve to the left (increased agonist potency). At this point, the EC_{50} is $\ll$ the K_{eq} for binding.

agonist will progressively shift to the left along the concentration axis. Figure 3.1 shows dose–response curves to a given agonist in a range of tissues of varying sensitivity (from low to high). It can be seen from this figure that the curves showing submaximal activity have similar EC_{50} values until the tissue maximal response is produced. Then, in the more sensitive tissues where full agonism is observed, the EC_{50} values progressively diminish (i.e., the curves shift to the left along the concentration axis).

The behavior of agonist dose–response curves in different tissues is important to understand in order to predict agonist response in all tissues. In general, in the least sensitive tissues, the dose–response curve to

any agonist emanates from concentrations around the K_{eq} for binding. At this point this will be denoted the K_A, which is the nomenclature for the binding K_{eq} for agonists. In more sensitive tissues, the curve shifts to the left of this value. Figure 3.2 shows the dose–response curves of two agonists (denoted A and B) in a range of tissues of varying sensitivity (numbered 1 to 4, with 1 being the most sensitive). In the lower panels the curves to each agonist in tissues 1 to 4 are shown. It can be seen that the relative potencies of agonists A and B do not follow a uniform pattern once partial agonism is observed. This has practical ramifications for drug discovery. Specifically, consider the relative potency profiles of agonists A and B in tissue 1 and tissue 4. In efficiently coupled

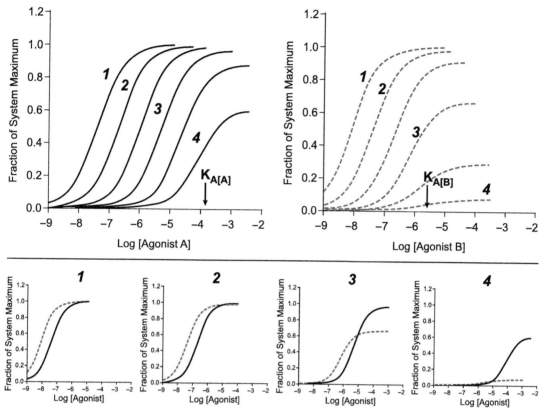

FIGURE 3.2 Dose–response curves to two agonists (Agonists A and B) in a range of systems of varying sensitivity. It can be seen that in systems of low sensitivity, both are partial agonists with potencies (EC$_{50}$ values) approximating the binding constant to the receptor (K$_{eq}$ for Agonist A = K$_{A[A]}$ and for Agonist B = K$_{A[B]}$). With increasing sensitivity, both become full agonists with increasing potency. Lower panels show the relative responses of each agonist in four systems ranked from most to least sensitive. It can be seen that the relative effects range from Agonist B being a more potent full agonist in system 1, to Agonist A being a more efficacious agonist in system 4. Thus, there is no uniform decrease and preservation of the relative activity of these agonists in the different systems due to the fact that agonist activity results from a complex interplay of affinity and efficacy.

tissues where both are full agonists, it can be seen that agonist B is more potent than agonist A. However, in a more poorly coupled tissue (tissue 4), it can be seen that agonist A now yields a more robust response than agonist B. Such discontinuities in agonist potency can only be predicted if the affinity and efficacy are known. In the absence of this information, the behavior of the agonists in different systems cannot be predicted accurately. The major

tool to make such predictions is the Black–Leff operational model of agonism.

NEW TERMINOLOGY

The following new terms will be introduced in this chapter:

- **Michaelis–Menten kinetics**: Description of the interaction of molecules with proteins based on the enzyme catalysis of substrate molecules as first described by Michaelis and Menten. Kinetics are characterized by a maximal rate of enzyme action (denoted **V_{max}**) and a sensitivity to catalysis (denoted **K_m**, referred to as the Michaelis–Menten constant). This latter term is the concentration of substrate that causes the enzyme to function at $\frac{1}{2} V_{max}$.

- **Receptor reserve (spare receptors)**: This refers to the condition in a tissue whereby the agonist needs to activate only a small fraction of the existing receptor population to produce the maximal system response. The magnitude of the reserve depends upon the sensitivity of the tissue *and* the efficacy of the agonist.
- **τ**: efficacy of an agonist (according to the Black–Leff operational model of agonism) made up of drug-specific properties (the intrinsic efficacy of the molecule) and tissue-related factors (the K_E of the drug-bound receptor interacting with the stimulus-response biochemical reactions of the cell).

THE BLACK–LEFF OPERATIONAL MODEL OF AGONISM

The model used to link the stimulus with cellular response is the operational model devised by Black and Leff.[1] The basis of this model is the experimental finding that the observed relationship between agonist-induced response and agonist concentration resembles a model of enzyme function presented in 1913 by Louis Michaelis and Maude L. Menten (see Box 3.1 and Fig. 3.3). This model accounts for the fact that the kinetics of enzyme reactions differ significantly from the kinetics of conventional chemical reactions. It describes the reaction of a substrate with an enzyme as an equation of the form: reaction velocity = (maximal velocity of the reaction × substrate concentration)/

(concentration of substrate + a fitting constant K_m). The parameter K_m characterizes the tightness of the binding of the reaction between the substrate and enzyme; it is also the concentration at which the reaction rate is half the maximal value. It can be seen that the more active the substrate, the smaller is the value of K_m. Comparison of this equation with equation 2.1 shows that it is formally identical to the Langmuir adsorption isotherm relating binding of a chemical to a surface ($K_m = K_{eq}$). Both of these models form the basis of drug receptor interaction, thus the kinetics involved sometimes are referred to as "Langmuirian" in form.

The Black–Leff model views the cell as a virtual enzyme and the amount of agonist–target bound complexes as the substrate for that enzyme (see Box 3.2). The first step in the response chain is the transduction of the activated receptor stimulus (quantified by the number of agonist–receptor complexes denoted [AR]) into cellular response. The number of [AR] complexes is given by the fraction of the receptor population bound by agonist (ρ_A given by the Langmuir adsorption isotherm, equation 2.1) multiplied by the number of receptors on the cell surface (denoted [R_t]; [AR] = $\rho_A \bullet$ [R_t]). The operational model relates tissue response to a Michaelis–Menten type of equation of the form:

$$\text{Response} = \frac{[AR]E_m}{[AR] + K_E} \quad (3.1)$$

where [AR] is the concentration of the amount of agonist-activated receptor, E_m is the maximal response that the system is able to produce under saturating stimulation (as the V_{max} in the Michaelis–Menten enzyme reaction) and K_E is the equilibrium dissociation constant of the activated receptor and response element (cellular machinery that responds to the activated receptor to generate cellular response) complex. The similarity between a standard pharmacological dose–response curve and

BOX 3.1

MICHAELIS–MENTEN ENZYME KINETICS

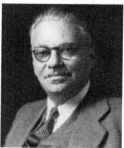
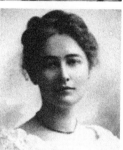

Leonor Michaelis (1875–1949) and Maude Menten (1879–1960) worked in the Berlin Municipal Hospital and together formulated one of the earliest quantitative laws of biochemistry. Specifically, their famous equation described the velocity and mechanism of the formation of the complex between an enzyme and substrate. In form, the Michaelis–Menten equation describes a relationship between input and output that is applicable to a wide variety of biochemical processes such as enzymes, transport processes and other saturable reactions. Black and Leff utilized the general form of this equation to define τ as a representation of agonist efficacy and the sensitivity of tissues to agonist action.

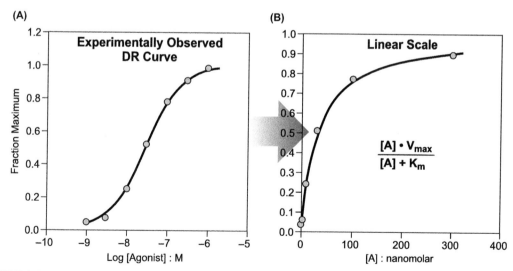

FIGURE 3.3 Similarity of cellular response to enzymatic function. Experimentally determined dose–response curve from an intact cell system (left panel) and the same curve plotted on a linear scale to show the similarity of the shape of this curve to a Michaelis–Menten kinetic system (right panel). This similarity prompted Black and Leff to use Michaelis–Menten kinetics to model cellular transduction of drug response.

BOX 3.2

THE OPERATIONAL MODEL OF DRUG ACTION ("SHOEBOX MODEL")

Stephenson's concept of efficacy was empirical in nature with no mechanistic basis. Black and Leff considered this to be a weakness in receptor theory and set out to redefine efficacy in biochemical terms as a function of a saturable transduction mechanism capable of being described with the Michaelis−Menten function for enzyme action. This model is rooted in what was observed in pharmacological experiments, namely that there is a hyperbolic relationship between agonist receptor occupancy and tissue response. An early version of the operational model was referred to by its creators as the "shoebox model" because of the fact that a three-dimensional rendering of the curves for agonist occupancy, signal transduction and end organ dose−response (as pasted on the internal faces of a shoebox) gave a concise view of the relationships between receptor occupancy and cellular response.

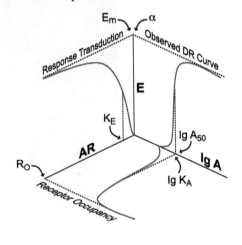

Michaelis−Menten kinetics is shown in Fig. 3.3. In this sense, equation 3.1 treats the cell as a comprehensive virtual enzyme utilizing the activated receptor as the substrate and cellular response as the product. The magnitude of the K_E reflects the activating power of the agonist, i.e., high efficacy agonists will have a lower K_E value than low efficacy agonists. The amount of [AR] complex is given by the Langmuir adsorption isotherm for the fractional receptor occupancy of the agonist (ρ_A from equation 2.1) to yield [AR] from $[AR] = \rho_A \bullet [R_t]$ where $[R_t]$ is the concentration of receptors. Combining equation 2.1 and the Michaelis−Menten equation (see Fig. 3.4 and Derivations and Proofs, Appendix B3):

$$\text{Response} = \frac{[A]/K_A[R_t]/K_E E_m}{[A]/K_A([R_t]/K_E + 1) + 1} \quad (3.2)$$

where E_m is the maximal response of the system. The model defines a parameter τ as $[R_t]/K_E$ to present the description of agonist response as:

$$\text{Response} = \frac{[A] \cdot \tau \cdot E_m}{[A](\tau + 1) + K_A} \quad (3.3)$$

An important and versatile parameter in the operational equation is τ; this constant incorporates the intrinsic efficacy of the agonist (a property of the molecule) and elements describing the efficiency of the tissue as it converts agonist-derived stimulus into tissue response (receptor density and K_E, the constant relating receptor activation and cellular response). The magnitude of K_E is unique for each tissue since it is an amalgam of the series of biochemical reactions unique to the cell.

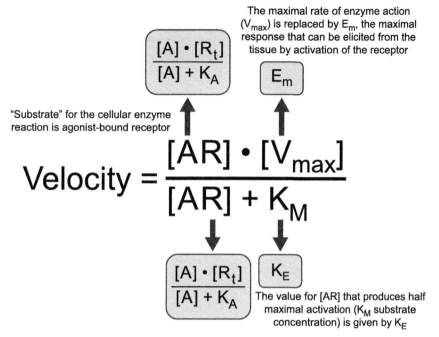

FIGURE 3.4 Operational model counterparts of the parameters of the Michaelis–Menten equation. Modeling cellular response as an enzyme velocity characterized by the Michaelis–Menten equation, the "substrate" for the cell is the agonist–receptor complex ([AR]) (given by the Langmuir adsorption isotherm). The sensitivity of the cell to agonist activation is quantified by K_E, while the maximal response of the system is denoted E_m.

APPLYING THE BLACK–LEFF MODEL TO PREDICT AGONISM

The first step in predicting agonism is to fit experimental data to the Black–Leff model; the variable slope version of the Black–Leff equation (see Derivations and Proofs, Appendix B4) should be used to accommodate varying dose–response curve slopes observed experimentally (see Box 3.3). There are three basic steps in this process; the first is to define the maximal response capability of the system (E_m) and estimate n, the slope factor of the dose–response curve. If a series of agonists all yield the same observed maximal response in a given preparation, this generally supports the postulate that the common observed maximal response is a reasonable estimate of E_m (it would be likely that all of the agonists are full agonists yielding the maximal response of the system). The slope of the dose–response curve can be obtained by independent fitting of the adsorption isotherm with no required added data (see Box 3.3). The second step is to obtain an estimate of K_A; if the ligands are partial agonists, then the EC_{50} (obtained from step 1) can be used as a first estimate of K_A to subsequently use for the computer fitting of data to the Black–Leff equation (for variable n; see Box 3.3). For a full agonist, the K_A must be estimated to some value greater than EC_{50}. The third is to fit the data to the model equation (see Fig. 3.5).

For high efficacy full agonists (high τ values), the maximal response will reflect the point at which the agonist saturates the

BOX 3.3

FITTING DOSE–RESPONSE DATA TO THE BLACK–LEFF MODEL

Under the correct circumstances, experimental dose–response data may be fit to the Black–Leff operational model to yield estimates of affinity (K_A) and efficacy (τ) for any agonist. Two essential parameters for this process are an independent estimate of E_m and an estimate of the affinity of the agonist; this latter parameter can be easily determined for a partial agonist as it will be approximated by the EC_{50}. The data is then fit to the simple adsorption isotherm to determine the slope of the curve (n):

$$\text{Response} = \frac{[A]^n \text{Max}}{[A]^n + EC_{50}^n}$$

These procedures will yield three of the four parameters necessary to start fitting to the equation for the Black–Leff model for all slopes of dose–response curve. This equation is:

$$\text{Response} = \frac{[A]^n \tau^n E_m}{[A]^n \tau^n + ([A] + K_A)^n}$$

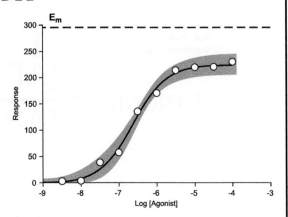

Least squares fitting by computer then yields a better estimate of K_A and a value for efficacy (τ), thereby completing the determination of all parameters needed to predict efficacy in other tissues.

stimulus–response capability of the cell and not the 100% receptor occupancy point. In fact there are numerous cell systems where powerful high efficacy agonists produce 100% maximal tissue response by occupying only a small fraction of the available receptors. Once the maximal tissue response is attained, occupancy of the remaining receptors by the agonist only serves to make the agonist more potent (i.e., the concentration–response curve shifts to the left along the concentration axis). For high efficacy agonists where the maximal cellular response can be obtained with a low level of receptor occupancy, the receptors occupied beyond the point where the maximum is attained are referred to as being "spare" (also

referred to as "receptor reserve" or "spare receptor capacity"). The maximal response of most tissues to powerful natural agonists (neurotransmitters, hormones) is produced by partial activation of the total receptor population on the cell surface; the remaining receptors appear to be "spare" and in fact participate in making the tissue more or less sensitive to the agonist. For example, the ileum of guinea pigs produces a maximal force of isometric contraction to the natural agonist histamine by activation of only 3% of the available receptors.[2] Therefore, in practical terms, 97% of the receptor population can be removed or inactivated with no decrease in the maximal response to histamine (albeit there is a loss in the

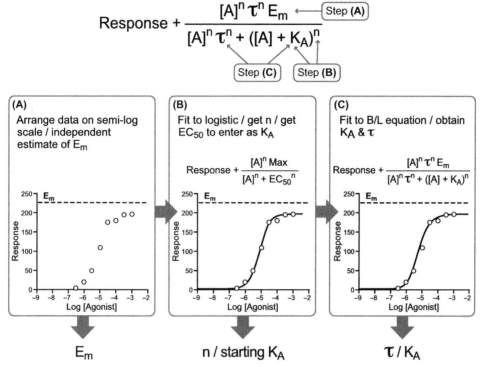

$$\text{Response} + \frac{[A]^n \tau^n E_m}{[A]^n \tau^n + ([A] + K_A)^n}$$ ← Step (A), Step (C), Step (B)

(A) Arrange data on semi-log scale / independent estimate of E_m

E_m

(B) Fit to logistic / get n / get EC_{50} to enter as K_A

$$\text{Response} + \frac{[A]^n \text{Max}}{[A]^n + EC_{50}^n}$$

n / starting K_A

(C) Fit to B/L equation / obtain K_A & τ

$$\text{Response} + \frac{[A]^n \tau^n E_m}{[A]^n \tau^n + ([A] + K_A)^n}$$

τ / K_A

FIGURE 3.5   Fitting the Black–Leff operational model to data. Step A arranges the data on a semi-logarithmic scale for response (versus dose of agonist); a maximal response of the system must be identified or assumed. Step B fits the data to a simple logistic function to yield the slope of the curve (n) and a measure of the location parameter along the concentration axis (EC_{50}). Step C then refits the data to the Black–Leff equation (shown at the top of the figure) using the predetermined values of E_m, n and estimating the K_A as the EC_{50} (in cases where the agonist is a partial agonist). In cases where the agonist is a full agonist, a value higher than the EC_{50} is used. This procedure yields an estimate of the efficacy (τ).

sensitivity to histamine). The term "receptor reserve" has been historically associated with the tissue (it involves the number of receptors in a given tissue and the efficiency with which they are coupled to the stimulus–response machinery of the cell). However, the intrinsic efficacy of the agonist is intimately involved in the magnitude of receptor reserve. Thus, the magnitude of the receptor reserve for two different agonists will be different; the agonist with the higher efficacy will have a greater receptor reserve, i.e., one agonist's spare receptor is a weaker agonist's essential one.

The major application of the Black–Leff operational model is the prediction of agonism in tissues. Specifically, the *ratio* of efficacies of two agonists (as ratios of τ values) is a *tissue-independent* measure of relative efficacy which can be measured in one test tissue and applied to all tissues. This is an important aspect of experimental pharmacology, as drugs are almost always tested and developed in one type of system for use in another (i.e., the therapeutic one). Reliance on tissue-dependent measures of drug activity (i.e., pEC_{50}, maximal response) is capricious and difficult to apply to the therapeutic environment without a tool such as the operational model to negate the effects of tissue type.

In general, once the ratio of τ and K_A values are defined for two agonists in one system, and assuming that the mechanism of response production for both agonists is the same; then these ratios can define the relative responses to those agonists in any tissue. There are a few key pieces of data required for this process. This will be illustrated with two hypothetical agonists, Agonist A (a reference standard) and Agonist B (a new test agonist). The first requirement is that the test system must be suitable to yield dose–response curves to both agonists (see Fig. 3.6, Panel 1); the Black–Leff operational

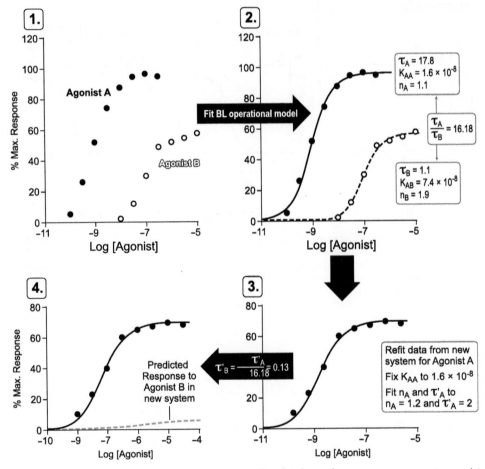

FIGURE 3.6 Measuring the relative efficacy of two agonists. Panel 1 shows dose–response curves to agonists A and B. The Black–Leff operational model is fit to these data points (see Fig. 3.5) to yield estimates of τ and K_A for each agonist. The ratio of the τ values should be a molecular system-independent parameter unique to the agonists. Panel 3 shows data in another system for one of the agonists. This is fit to the Black–Leff model to yield a τ value for this system. It will be assumed that the τ for the second agonist will adhere to the ratio of τ values found in the first system. This predicts that the τ for the second agonist in this system will be 0.13. The predicted response to Agonist B is obtained by back-calculating response according to the Black–Leff model with the designated K_A and τ values.

model is fit to the data to yield estimates of K_A and τ for each agonist (Fig. 3.6, Panel 2). From this procedure, a ratio for τ_A/τ_B is obtained; this is a molecular property that is unique to both of these agonists and links agonism produced by each in any system. The next requirement is that a dose–response curve be obtained in the system for which the prediction will be made; the assumption is that the curve for the reference agonist (Agonist A) is observed in this system (Fig. 3.6, Panel 3). The Black–Leff model is fit to the data for the reference agonist in this system. It is assumed that the affinity of the agonist will be the same in the test system and this new system. With this procedure, a new τ'_A value is obtained. Then, using the affinity for the test agonist (Agonist B) obtained from the test

system and a predicted efficacy τ'_B equal to $\tau_B \times$ the ratio of efficacies for the two agonists calculated in the test system (τ_A/τ_B), a predicted new efficacy for Agonist B is used in the Black–Leff equation to predict the responses to agonist B in the new system (Fig. 3.6, Panel 4). In the particular example shown it is seen that little response to the test agonist would be predicted from the calculated ratio of efficacies (τ_A/τ_B) estimated in the test system.

This is a powerful tool to predict agonism that has value in predicting *in vivo* activity from *in vitro* data. Assuming that the pharmacokinetics of the agonists are adequate to yield exposure of the target to the agonists *in vivo* (see Chapters 7 and 8), predictions using the Black–Leff operational model can detect test

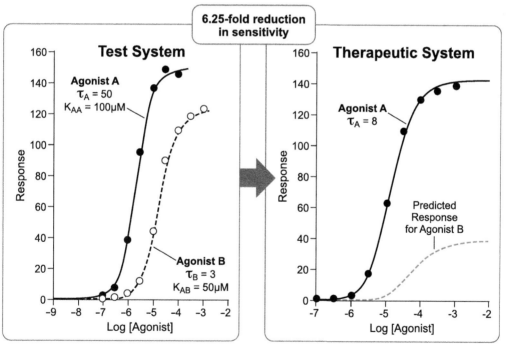

FIGURE 3.7 Prediction of relative responses to agonists in a therapeutic system 6.25-fold less sensitive than the test system. The relative τ values for Agonists A and B were found to be $\tau_A/\tau_B = 16.7$ (left panel). The curve to Agonist A furnishes the τ for the system in the right panel, indicating the 6.25 decrease in sensitivity. Thus the τ values for Agonist B divided by this ratio predict the τ in that system to predict the curve of Agonist B (broken line).

agonists that would not warrant testing in high resource *in vivo* assays. For example, Fig. 3.7 shows data for a reference agonist (Agonist A) and a test Agonist B ($\tau_A/\tau_B = 5/0.3 = 16.7$). Testing of the reference Agonist A in the *in vivo* system showed that a 6.25-fold loss of sensitivity occurs from testing in the *in vitro* test system compared to the *in vivo* system. Assuming comparable pharmacokinetics (an important assumption), the Black–Leff operational model predicts that considerably less agonism will be observed in the *in vivo* system with Agonist B.

This result is intuitively obvious from the profile of these agonists since it is clear that Agonist B is less efficacious and potent than Agonist A in the test system. Specifically, it is clear that a 6.25-fold loss of sensitivity in the systems would impact Agonist B more than Agonist A in terms of observed agonism. However, the power of this method extends beyond such obvious predictions. As seen in Fig. 3.2, the response to an agonist becomes depressed as the concentrations approach the K_A. Therefore, in cases where the affinity of the test agonist is higher than the affinity of the reference agonist, but the efficacy is lower, surprising profiles can result in systems of lowered sensitivity. Figure 3.8 shows a system whereby the test agonist is actually more potent than the reference agonist. However, this increased potency is due to a higher affinity, not a higher

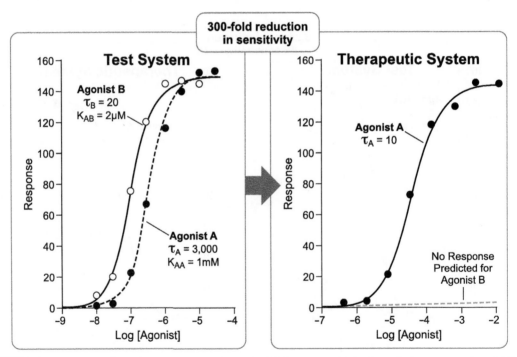

FIGURE 3.8   Prediction of agonism in a system after a 300-fold loss in sensitivity from the test system. Agonist B has a higher affinity but lower efficacy than Agonist A. Nevertheless, the higher affinity causes Agonist B to be more potent than Agonist A in the test system. However, in the 300-fold less sensitive system, the low efficacy of Agonist B prevents any agonism being observed, so there is a striking reversal of effects with Agonist A being more active than Agonist B. This type of reversal could not be predicted without quantifying the relative affinities and efficacies of the two agonists.

efficacy ($\tau_A/\tau_B = 150$). Therefore, in an *in vivo* system where the reference Agonist A is 1/300 as active, the surprising prediction that the response to Agonist B will disappear is made from application of the Black–Leff operational model (see Fig. 3.8).

DESCRIPTIVE PHARMACOLOGY: III

Continuing the theme of a progressive characterization of the drug effect of molecules through pharmacologic procedures, Fig. 3.9 shows the next step in quantifying observed full or partial agonism. Specifically, estimation of the affinity and relative affinity of a test agonist theoretically could lead to the ability to predict agonism to that test agonist in any system. At this time it should be stressed that there are two overriding assumptions in this procedure. The first is that the concentrations used on the abscissa axis of the dose–response curves (whether *in vitro* or *in vivo*) accurately reflect the concentration present at the target interface. The second is that the mechanism of action of the test and reference agonists in producing a response is identical. If either of these assumptions is not true, then dissimulations between predicted and observed agonism will occur.

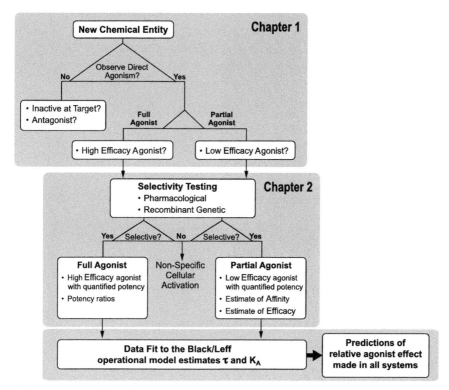

FIGURE 3.9 Continuation of logical progression for determination of new drug effect (from Fig. 2.11). Agonist dose–response curves are fit to the Black–Leff operational model to yield estimates of affinity (K_A) and efficacy (τ). These can be used to predict agonism in other systems.

SUMMARY

- The sensitivity of cells to directly activating molecules (agonists) depends upon intrinsic properties of the molecule (affinity and intrinsic efficacy) and the cell system (receptor number and efficiency of receptor coupling). The operational model allows ascription of molecular properties (affinity in the form of K_A and efficacy in the form of τ); this model allows prediction of agonist effect in different tissues from ratios of K_A and τ obtained for agonists.

QUESTIONS

3.1 Why did Black and Leff use the Michaelis–Menten equation as the basis for signal transduction in the operational model?

3.2 Describe how the operational model parameter τ characterizes both the intrinsic efficacy of the agonist and the sensitivity of the system.

3.3 A given agonist A was found to have a receptor reserve of 90% in a given tissue system. What does this mean? Another agonist B had a reserve in the same tissue of only 40%; what properties of agonists A and B could lead to this result?

References

[1] J.W. Black, P. Leff, Operational models of pharmacological agonist, Proc. R. Soc. Lond. [Biol.] 220 (1983) 141.
[2] M. Nickerson, Receptor occupancy and tissue response, Nature 178 (1956) 697–698.

4

Drug Antagonism: Orthosteric Drug Effects

By the end of this chapter readers should be able to quantify the effects of antagonists to yield empirical measures of antagonist potency. They will also be able to relate patterns of antagonism produced by orthosteric antagonists (those producing steric hindrance of agonists) to mechanisms of antagonist action. Readers will then be able to use these mechanisms to apply the appropriate mathematical analysis to yield estimates of true system-independent antagonist potency that transcend cell type and measuring system.

BI-MOLECULAR SYSTEMS

The previous chapters discussed the binding of a molecule to a protein target to cause a change in cellular function (agonism); in these cases the system consists of a single molecule interacting with a target on the cell. There are a large number of pharmacologically relevant interactions that involve *two molecules*; one causing a change of cellular function and the other interfering with that action. For example, Fig. 4.1 shows a synaptic cleft where a

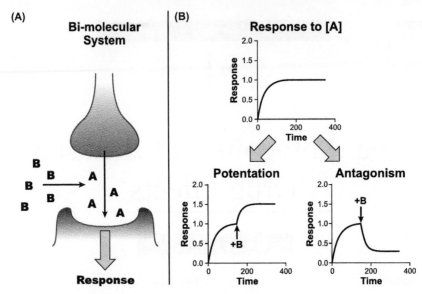

FIGURE 4.1 Schematic diagram of a physiological system consisting of a neuron releasing an agonist A and the addition of an external compound B. If B has an affinity for the target, the response to A can be increased (potentiated) or blocked. Potentiation would be an allosteric mechanism (discussed in Chapter 5); antagonism is the subject of this present chapter.

neurotransmitter molecule A is released from the neuron to act on the post-synaptic membrane containing receptors for that neurotransmitter; molecule B can be added to the system to modify the interaction of A with the target. There are two pharmacologically relevant outcomes, namely that the response to A can be increased or diminished (see Fig. 4.1). If the response is increased this could be due to an interference in the disposition of A in the synaptic cleft (inhibition of transport) or allosteric alteration of the target to increase responsiveness. This latter topic will be discussed in Chapter 5. This present chapter discusses the inhibition of the response to A. Implicit in this discussion is the understanding that the effects seen are specific for the drug target being considered, i.e., the molecule does not produce non-specific toxic or other effects on the cell system to modify the cell sensitivity to the agonist.

NEW TERMINOLOGY

The following new terms will be introduced in this chapter:

- **Allosteric**: Describing an interaction mediated by the binding of a molecule to a protein at a distinct site to affect the interaction of that protein with another molecule binding at a different site.
- **Antagonism:** The process of inhibition of an agonist-driven cellular response by another molecule.
- **Competitive antagonism**: A specific model of receptor antagonism whereby two molecules compete for a single binding site on the receptor, and the kinetics of binding of both the agonist and antagonist are rapid enough to allow mass action to control the relative proportions of receptor bound to agonist and antagonist.

- **Hemi-equilibrium**: A condition where there is an insufficient amount of time for complete re-equilibration of agonist and antagonist for a population of receptors according to mass action. This results in a selectively non-competitive effect at high agonist receptor occupancies, causing a partial depression of the maximal response to the agonist.
- **Insurmountable**: Describing a pattern of agonist dose−response curves whereby the maximal response to the agonist is depressed.
- **Non-competitive**: Describing antagonism resulting from a system whereby the antagonist does not dissociate from the receptor rapidly enough to allow competition with the agonist.
- **Orthosteric**: A steric interaction whereby molecules compete for binding at the same site on a protein.
- **pA$_2$**: Minus logarithm of the molar concentration of an antagonist that produces a two-fold shift of the agonist dose−response curve.
- **pIC$_{50}$**: Minus logarithm of the molar concentration of antagonist that produces a 50% inhibition of a defined agonist effect.
- **pK$_B$**: Minus logarithm of the equilibrium dissociation constant of the antagonist−receptor complex.
- **Schild analysis**: The application of the Schild equation to a set of dextral displacements produced by a surmountable antagonist; if the Schild plot is linear with a slope of unity the antagonism fulfills criteria for simple competitive antagonism.
- **Surmountable**: Describing antagonism whereby the agonist dose−response curve is shifted to the right with increasing addition of antagonist, but where the maximal response is not altered.

WHAT IS DRUG ANTAGONISM?

This chapter will deal with molecules that bind to the target without themselves causing a change (or producing relatively little change), but do interfere with agonists producing response; this is the process of *antagonism*. There are many therapeutically relevant conditions where an antagonist would be useful, as in cases of inappropriate, excessive or persistent agonism (i.e., inflammation, gastric ulcer) or diseases where remodeling of systems leads to normal agonism becoming harmful (cardiovascular disease). Conceptually, antagonism could be envisioned as the binding of the antagonist to a target to hinder the binding or function (or both) of an agonist. There are three factors that control the extent of antagonism:

- the quantity of antagonist bound (**potency**);
- the location of the binding relative to the binding of the natural agonist (**mechanism**);
- the persistence of antagonist binding (**antagonist kinetics**).

It is worth considering each of these important factors when discussing therapeutically relevant antagonism.

ANTAGONIST POTENCY

Potency refers to the amount of antagonism in a system for a given concentration of antagonist. The relevant parameter for this is the affinity of the antagonist for the protein target (as defined by Langmuir adsorption binding isotherm; see equation 2.1). Unlike agonism, estimates of antagonist potency should not be cell-type dependent, and thus these are chemical terms that can be measured in a test system and the result applied to all systems, including the therapeutic one. The affinity of an antagonist, quantified as the equilibrium dissociation constant of the antagonist—protein complex, can be measured in an appropriate *in vitro* system either directly (if a means to trace the protein-bound antagonist species can be quantified, such as in radiolabeled binding assays) or indirectly through interference of agonist activity in a functional assay. This latter approach is preferable as it is what the antagonist will do *in vivo* that is important. In addition, there are numerous cases where physical binding of molecules and their effect on physiological responses can differ. The desired parameter in this case is referred to as the pK_B, namely the negative logarithm of the equilibrium dissociation constant of the antagonist—protein complex. To measure antagonist potency in an *in vitro* functional assay, comparisons are made between the dose—response curve of the agonist produced in the absence of antagonist, and then again in the presence of antagonist (usually for a range of antagonist concentrations). The resulting pattern of curves is then utilized in an appropriate model defined by the proposed mechanism of action of the antagonist. It should be noted that the antagonism must be shown to be specific for the biological target in question (see Fig. 4.2); it will be assumed that the observed antagonist effects are specific for the target.

There are two effects an antagonist can have on the dose—response curve to an agonist: depression of maximal response and dextral displacement of the curve (or both; see Fig. 4.3). Both of these effects reflect a diminution of the sensitivity of the system to the agonist in the presence of the antagonist, thus higher concentrations of agonist are required to produce a response in the presence of the antagonist. Different mechanisms of antagonism can produce varying amounts of shift and depression of maxima of the dose—response curves. This can also vary with the type of agonist used to produce response and the sensitivity of the functional system used to measure the effect. For this reason, the pattern(s) of antagonism seen *in vitro* cannot reliably be used to identify the mechanism of action; in fact, the reverse is true. Once a mechanism of action is identified, then the appropriate model is applied to the data to characterize antagonist potency (pK_B values).

MECHANISM(S) OF RECEPTOR ANTAGONISM

There are two molecular mechanisms operable for the antagonism of responses to

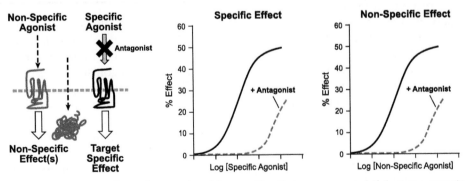

FIGURE 4.2 Determining specificity of antagonism. Non-specific effects are suggested if the test antagonist blocks the effect of a non-specific stimulant of the cell (i.e., acting through another receptor or otherwise elevating response biochemically).

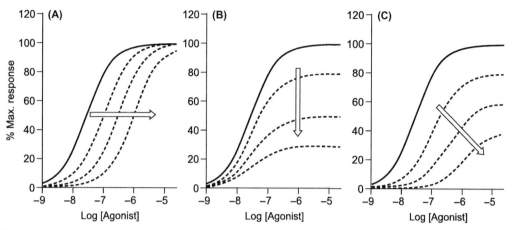

FIGURE 4.3 Orthosteric target antagonism can take the form of a shift to the right of the agonist dose–response curve (A), a depression of the maximal response to the agonist (B) or a mixture of the two effects.

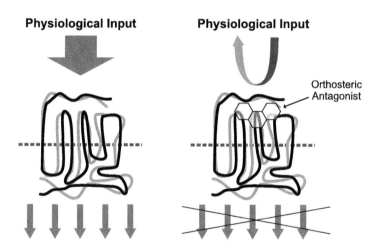

FIGURE 4.4 Orthosteric antagonism prevents the binding of the agonist to the target active binding site. Under these circumstances all functions mediated by the target, as a result of agonist binding, will be blocked.

endogenous hormones, neurotransmitters or autacoids: orthosteric or allosteric binding. Orthosteric antagonism (see Fig. 4.4) is where the antagonist binds to the same site as the endogenous agonist and precludes agonist binding to the protein. This mechanism is preemptive, in that occupancy of the site by the antagonist prevents all actions of the agonist. The second mechanism (allosteric; see Fig. 4.5) is where the antagonist and agonist bind to separate binding sites on the protein, and the interaction between them occurs through a change in conformation of the protein. This type of mechanism is permissive in that some (or even all) actions of the agonist can still be produced when the antagonist is bound. However, some characteristics of the agonist response are modified, such as potency and/ or efficacy. Orthosteric antagonism is the most simple and will be discussed in this present chapter; allosteric mechanisms will be discussed in Chapter 5.

Physiological Input   **Physiological Input**

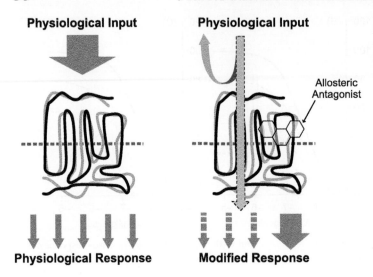

Allosteric
Antagonist

Physiological Response   **Modified Response**

FIGURE 4.5 Allosteric interactions are permissive in that both the probe molecule (agonist, radioligand) and the allosteric modulator bind to the protein simultaneously and the modulator may allow some or all of the probe molecule effects to be observed. The example shown above is for an allosteric antagonist; therefore the resulting agonist effect may be partially or completely blocked.

ORTHOSTERIC (COMPETITIVE AND NON-COMPETITIVE) ANTAGONISM

As discussed in Chapter 2, the binding of a molecule to a protein is a stochastic process, meaning that at any one instant there will be a population of protein binding sites where the antagonist is tightly bound to the protein and another where it has momentarily diffused away from the binding site, leaving it open for binding to other molecules. Thus, the probability of another molecule (e.g., agonist) binding to the same site in the presence of the antagonist will be determined by the amount of time the antagonist is momentarily not bound to the protein (determined in turn by the affinity and concentration of the antagonist), and the concentration and affinity of the agonist. Thus it can be seen that in such a system of competition, a very high concentration of agonist theoretically could bind to all of the sites and the maximal response to the agonist would be attained even in the presence of the antagonist. This idea is captured in a simple equation presented by John Gaddum (see Box 4.1), known as the Gaddum equation for competitive

kinetics. Specifically, this equation relates the fractional receptor occupancy by a molecule A (ρ_A) to the concentration A (denoted c_A, referring to the concentration normalized as a fraction of the equilibrium dissociation constant of the A−receptor complex), and the normalized concentration of another drug B competing for the same site on the receptor (see Derivations and Proofs, Appendix B5):[1]

$$\rho_A = \frac{C_A}{1 + C_A + C_B} \quad (4.1)$$

Therefore, in a completely competitive situation, where the binding of both the antagonist and agonist are rapid, the dose−response curve to the agonist will be shifted to the right in the presence of the competitive antagonist and very high concentrations of agonist will produce the original maximal response (obtained in the absence of antagonist) even in the presence of the antagonist. The shift to the right of the agonist curve reflects the lower probability of the agonist producing a response in the presence of the obstructing antagonist; this probability is increased with increased agonist concentration, therefore the curve reappears at higher concentrations of

---

BOX 4.1

THE GADDUM EQUATION

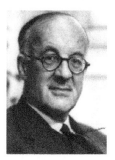

Sir John Gaddum (1900–1965)

John Henry Gaddum (1900–1965) was a British pharmacologist who did a great deal to propagate quantitative pharmacology. Educated at Cambridge, Gaddum became a medical student at University College London where he applied for, and won, a post at the Wellcome Research Laboratories. There he wrote his first paper on quantitative drug antagonism. After working for the influential pharmacologist Sir Henry Hallet Dale and later chairing the Department of Pharmacology at Cairo University,

Gaddum returned to University College London to head the Department of Pharmacology there. At this time, he presented a short communication to the Physiological Society in 1937 entitled "The quantitative effects of antagonistic drugs"[1] which contained the famous "Gaddum equation:"

$$\rho_A = \frac{C_A}{1 + C_A + C_B}$$

where ρ_A is the fractional receptor occupancy by drug A in the presence of another drug B that competes for the binding of A at the receptor. The terms c_A and c_B refer to the normalized (divided by the equilibrium dissociation constants of the drug–receptor complexes) concentrations of a drugs A and B respectively. It can be seen that if $c_A \gg c_B$, then the total occupancy of the receptor will revert to a situation identical to that where only molecule A is present, i.e., it will compete with B to the extent that B no longer occupies the receptor.

---

agonist. The magnitude of the shift in the dose–response curve is proportional to the degree of antagonism and relates to the concentration of antagonist present and its affinity. Schild and colleagues (see Box 4.2) used this fact to devise a method to measure the affinity of competitive antagonists, in a procedure since given the name "Schild analysis" for the construction of a "Schild plot."[2] The procedure for doing this is shown in Fig. 4.6. The first step is to define the sensitivity of the system to the agonist (obtain a control dose–response curve). Then, the preparation is pre-equilibrated with a defined

concentration of the antagonist; this ensures that the receptors and antagonist come to a binding equilibrium according to the Langmuir isotherm. Then, the sensitivity of the tissue is measured again in the presence of the pre-equilibrated antagonist and the shift in the curve is used to estimate the antagonist potency.

For Schild analysis, this is done repeatedly with a range of antagonist concentrations, and then an array of shifts of the control curve produced by a matching array of antagonist concentrations is used to estimate the affinity of the antagonist. The shifts are quantified as

---

BOX 4.2

H. O. SCHILD AND THE "SCHILD EQUATION"

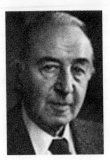

Heinz Schild (1906–1984)

Heinz Schild took Gaddum's equation for competitive binding and ingeniously extended it to provide a tool for the measurement of the potency of a competitive antagonist blocking agonist response. The key to this is the application of the null assumption stating that equal responses to an agonist emanate from equal levels of receptor occupancy by that agonist. This allows the response to a concentration of an agonist A (c_A), measured in the absence of

an antagonist B, to be represented by ρ_A. This is the receptor occupancy by A, as given by the Gaddum equation, to be represented (since equal responses are being compared) by the response of the same agonist obtained in the presence of the antagonist:

$$\rho_A = \frac{C_A}{1 + C_A} = \frac{C_A'}{1 + C_A' + C_B}$$

The concentration of agonist in this latter situation (denoted c_A') will be greater in the presence of the antagonist since it must overcome the competition by antagonist. Cross multiplication and dividing the entire expression by c_A results in the Schild equation where c_A'/c_A is denoted by the equiactive dose–ratio DR:

Schild Equation

$$\frac{C_A'}{C_A} = C_B + 1 = \frac{[B]}{K_B} + 1 = DR$$

---

ratios of the EC_{50} of the agonist in the presence and absence of antagonist; these are referred to as dose ratios ($DR = EC_{50[antagonist]}/EC_{50[control]}$). It can be shown that the $\log(DR - 1)$ values for a range of concentrations of antagonist [B] have a linear relationship according to the "Schild equation" (see Box 4.2):

$$\text{Log}(DR - 1) = \text{Log}[B] - pK_B \qquad (4.2)$$

where pK_B is the negative logarithm of the equilibrium dissociation constant of the antagonist–receptor complex; this parameter is a system-independent measure of the potency of a competitive antagonist. An example of this type of analysis is given in Fig. 4.7. It should

be noted that for there to be confidence in the veracity of pK_B as a true measure of antagonist potency, the Schild plot (line according to equation 4.2) should be linear and have a slope of unity.

At this point it is worth discussing another practical method of quantifying the potency of competitive and indeed nearly any other kind of, antagonist. As discussed in Chapter 1, the Langmuir adsorption isotherm shows that the concentration of antagonism equal to K_B (K_{eq} in the binding isotherm) occupies 50% of the receptor population. It can be shown that occupancy of 50% of the receptor population by the antagonist will necessitate a doubling of the

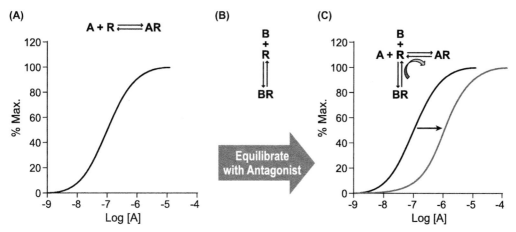

FIGURE 4.6 The process of assessing receptor antagonism. (A) The sensitivity of the system to the agonist is measured through observation of an agonist dose–response curve. (B) After the agonist is removed, the tissue is equilibrated with a given concentration of antagonist. (C) In the presence of the antagonist, the sensitivity to the agonist is again measured with an agonist dose–response curve.

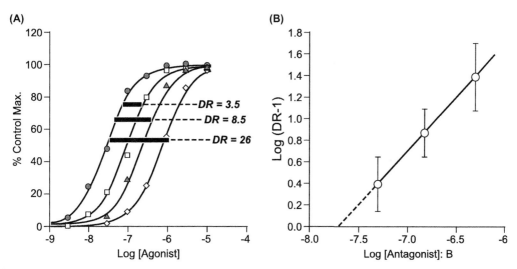

FIGURE 4.7 Schild analysis. (A) Dose–response curves to the agonist are obtained in the absence and presence of various concentrations of antagonist. The resulting shifts to the right of the agonist dose–response curves are converted to dose ratios (DR) and utilized in the Schild equation (equation 4.2) to construct a Schild regression (shown in panel (B)). Thus, a regression of Log(DR −1) values for a given array of antagonist concentrations provides a linear regression (ideally with a slope of unity) the intercept of which is − pK_B.

concentration of agonist to produce the same level of response obtained in the absence of antagonist. This means that in the presence of this concentration of antagonist, the dose ratio for the agonist will be 2. This can be seen from the Schild equation, where at DR = 2, Log [B] = − pK_B. The concentration that produces a two-fold shift to the right of the agonist dose—response curve is thus a characteristic measure of potency (being an estimate of the K_B or the concentration producing 50% receptor occupancy); it is referred to as the pA_2, specifically the negative logarithm of the molar concentration of antagonist that produces a two-fold shift to the right of the agonist dose—response curve. The pA_2 can readily be calculated by measuring the shift to the right produced by a single concentration of antagonist (as long as it is ≥ 2), and calculating the pA_2 through the relationship (see Box 4.3):

$$pA_2 = Log(DR - 1) - Log[B] \qquad (4.3)$$

In general, it is not prudent to simply obtain a pA_2 estimate and assume that it represents the true affinity as a pK_B; a complete Schild analysis allows observation of the criteria for true competitive inhibition, namely that the regression should be linear and have a slope of unity. If these conditions are not met, then the pA_2 is an empirical measure of antagonist potency which still can be of value, but may not equal the true pK_B.

Schild analysis was presented as a linear transform at a time where fitting data to models was more difficult than it is in the present day. An alternative to using the linearly transformed Schild analysis approach is to fit the raw data directly to the model for simple competitive antagonism. This is represented by an equation yielding the response to the agonist [A] in the presence of a concentration of antagonist [B] in the following form:

$$Response = \frac{([A]/EC_{50})^n \ Max}{([A]/EC_{50})^n + ([B]/K_B)^n + 1} \qquad (4.4)$$

BOX 4.3

ESTIMATION OF COMPETITIVE ANTAGONIST POTENCY THROUGH THE pA_2

In practical terms, all that is required to estimate the potency of a simple competitive antagonist is the determination of the effect of a single concentration of the antagonist on an agonist dose—response curve. As shown in the figure to the right, a control dose—response curve to an agonist (filled circles) is shifted to the right in the presence of a $1\,\mu M$ concentration of antagonist [B]; see curve denoted by open circles. The magnitude of the dose ratio (DR) is given by the ratio of the EC_{50} concentrations of agonist in the presence of antagonist (in this case 270 nM) and absence of antagonist (in this case 30 nM); thus for this example, DR = 270/30 = 9. According to the pA_2 calculation from equation 4.3 the pA_2 is:

$$pA_2 = Log(9 - 1) - Log(1\ \mu M) = 0.9 - (-6) = 6.9$$

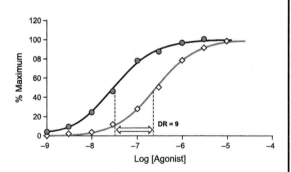

This is a unique estimate of this antagonist's potency, meaning that a molar concentration of $10^{-6.9} = 126$ nM shifts the dose—response curve by a factor of two and binds to 50% of the receptors in any tissue.

where n is the slope parameter for the agonist dose–response curve, Max is the maximal asymptote of the agonist dose–response curve, EC_{50} is the concentration of agonist producing the half-maximal response and K_B is the desired parameter, namely the equilibrium dissociation constant for the antagonist–receptor complex. An example of direct fitting of dose–response data to the competitive model is shown in Fig. 4.8.

Three methods of measuring the affinity of a competitive antagonist have been discussed: pA_2 as an empirical measure (equation 4.3); pK_B from Schild analysis (equation 4.2) and pK_B through direct fitting to equation 4.4. In all of these cases, no useful data can be obtained until the antagonist is present in the receptor compartment at a concentration that occupies $\geq 50\%$ of the receptors (this produces $DR = 2$). Lower concentrations than this will produce little change in the agonist dose–response curve and thus yield no data for calculation. When testing an antagonist of unknown potency, this poses a problem in terms of which concentration should first be

equilibrated with the preparation to yield useful data. For this reason, when unknown antagonists are to be tested, another strategy, namely determining the pIC_{50}, is used. This strategy pre-activates the system with agonist and then adds a range of concentrations of antagonist; then the resulting effect on the elevated basal response is measured. Figure 4.9 shows how pre-equilibration of the system with an EC_{50} of agonist yields an inverse sigmoidal curve which then can be used to estimate the pIC_{50}, namely the negative logarithm of the molar concentration of antagonist that reduces the agonist response by 50%. It can be seen that considerably fewer data points are required for this estimate. The pIC_{50} for a competitive antagonist then can be used to calculate the pK_B for the antagonist through a correction equation given as (see Derivations and Proofs, Appendix B6 [3]):

$$pK_B = -\text{Log}\left[\frac{IC_{50}}{((2 + ([A]/EC_{50})^n)^{1/n} - 1}\right] \quad (4.5)$$

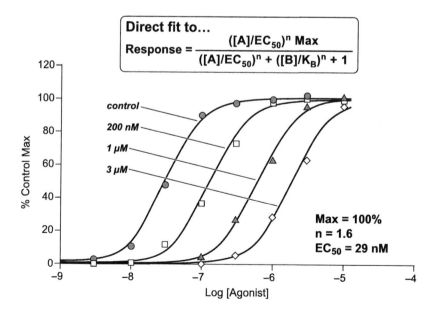

Direct fit to...

$$\text{Response} = \frac{([A]/EC_{50})^n \text{ Max}}{([A]/EC_{50})^n + ([B]/K_B)^n + 1}$$

Max = 100%
n = 1.6
EC_{50} = 29 nM

control
200 nM
1 µM
3 µM

% Control Max
Log [Agonist]

FIGURE 4.8 Direct fitting of data to the simple competitive model of antagonism (equation 4.4) to yield, in this case, a pK_B for the antagonist of 7.25.

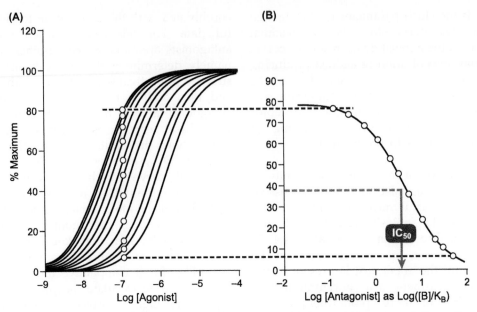

FIGURE 4.9 Effects of a simple competitive antagonist on an agonist dose–response curve (left panel); open circles show the effects of the antagonist on a selected dose of agonist that produces 80% maximal response in the absence of the antagonist. Right panel shows the responses to that same selected dose of agonist as a function of the concentrations of competitive antagonist producing the blockade. It can be seen that an inverse sigmoidal curve results (pIC$_{50}$ curve). The value of the abscissa corresponding to the half-maximal ordinate value of this curve is the IC$_{50}$, namely the molar concentration of antagonist that produces half-maximal inhibition of the defined agonist response.

It should be noted that equation 4.5 is valid only for those antagonists that produce surmountable antagonism; if the antagonism is insurmountable, then a different relationship will be operative between the pIC$_{50}$ and the pK$_B$ (*vide infra*).

SLOW DISSOCIATION KINETICS AND NON-COMPETITIVE ANTAGONISM

For true competitive kinetics to be operative, the antagonist that has been pre-equilibrated with the receptors must dissociate quickly enough for the agonist present in the receptor compartment to bind according to mass action (Fig. 4.10A). If this does not occur, the antagonist will occupy an inordinately high

percentage of the receptors and antagonism will dominate. This percentage of receptors could be high enough to prevent the agonist from producing a maximal response, thus an insurmountable effect on the agonist dose–response curve will result (Fig. 4.10B). This is sometimes also referred to as "pseudo-irreversible" antagonism, because the antagonist is essentially irreversibly bound to the receptor within the time-frame relevant for the production of response by the agonist. This often results in a depressed maximal response in the agonist dose–response curve. The degree of maximal response depression depends on the number of receptors needed to induce response in the cell preparation, i.e., the magnitude of the receptor reserve (see Chapter 3). If the cell is extremely sensitive to the agonist, such that only a small fraction of the receptor population

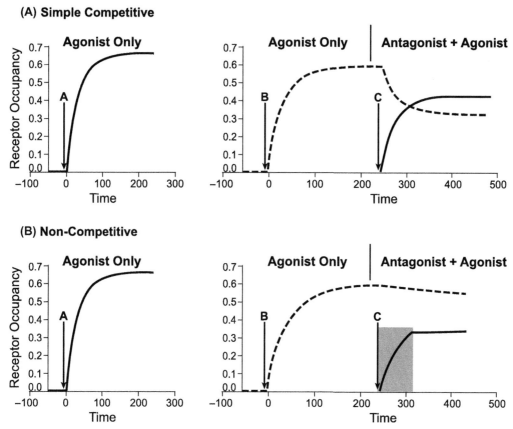

FIGURE 4.10   The kinetics of re-equilibration of agonists, antagonists and receptors. (A) For simple competitive antagonist systems where there is sufficient time for re-equilibration between receptors. The reduction in antagonist receptor occupancy (dotted line) rapidly adjusts as the agonist binds to receptors (solid line). (B) For a slowly dissociating antagonist (broken line), the agonist binding is biphasic, characterized by an initial rapid phase (where the agonist binds to open receptors) and a slow phase whereby the agonist must deal with a slowly dissociating antagonist. The gray rectangle represents the window of opportunity to measure agonist response in the presence of the antagonist; if this is less than the time required for complete re-equilibration of agonist, antagonist and receptors then the agonist receptor occupancy will be less than would be defined by true competitive interactions.

needs to be activated to produce tissue maximal response, then even an irreversible antagonist may shift the curve to the right with little depression of maximum, i.e., if only 7% of the receptors are needed for maximal response, then irreversibly blocking 80% of the receptors will still enable the agonist to produce a maximal response. On the other hand, if the cell is not very sensitive to the agonist and 100% of the receptors are needed for the production of maximal response, an irreversible antagonist will immediately produce a depression of the maximal response to the agonist. These different scenarios are shown in Fig. 4.11. In cases of true non-competitive orthosteric blockade where the maximal response to the agonist is depressed by all concentrations of antagonist, the pIC_{50} can be obtained as for competitive antagonists (Fig. 4.9)

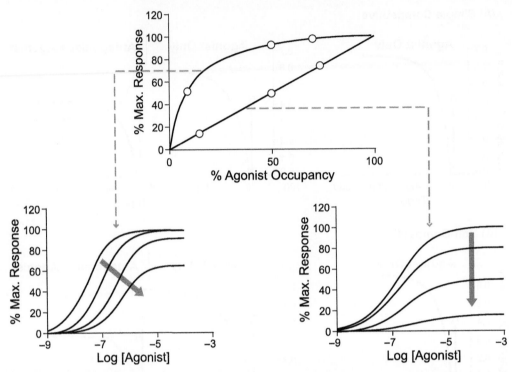

FIGURE 4.11   The effects of a non-competitive antagonist in two different tissue systems. The top left panel is a system possessing a receptor reserve for the agonist (100% response can be obtained by occupancy of 70% of the receptors). Therefore, non-competitive (pseudo-irreversible) blockade of receptors will result in dextral displacement of the agonist dose—response curve with no depression of maximal response until concentrations of antagonist that block >70% are present. The response system to the right has no reserve for the agonist (note the linear relationship between percentage agonist occupancy and response). Under these circumstances, the non-competitive antagonist will produce depression of the maximal response to the agonist at all concentrations.

and the resulting pIC_{50} is essentially equal to the pK_B (see Fig. 4.12). This obviates the use of a correction factor such as that provided by equation 4.5.

So far, two kinetic extremes of orthosteric antagonist action have been discussed; a rapidly dissociating antagonist that allows true competitiveness between agonist and antagonist to result and a slowly dissociating antagonist (essentially irreversible) that causes the antagonist to eliminate a certain fraction of the receptor from consideration of agonism. There are a large number of systems, referred to as "hemi-equilibria," that

fall in between these extremes. Here, the antagonist partially dissociates from the receptors in the presence of the agonist causing only the high concentrations of agonist (those requiring high receptor occupancies) to be subjected to irreversible blockade. Under these circumstances, the dose—response curves to the agonist are shifted to the right by the antagonist but may have a truncated (essentially "chopped") maximal response (see Fig. 4.13). In these cases, the potency of the antagonist can be estimated with a pA_2 and/or Schild analysis on the parallel shifted portions of the curves.

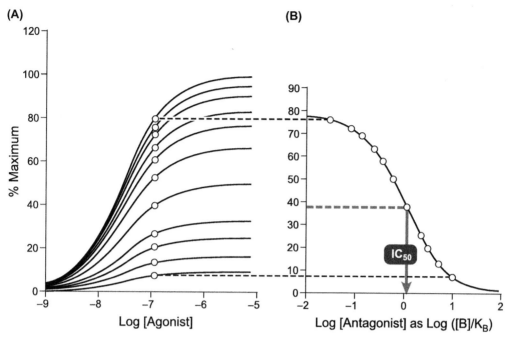

FIGURE 4.12   Effects of a non-competitive antagonist on an agonist dose–response curve (left panel); open circles show the effects of the antagonist on a selected dose of agonist that produces 80% maximal response in the absence of the antagonist. Right panel shows the responses to that same selected dose of agonist as a function of the concentrations of competitive antagonist producing the blockade. It can be seen that an inverse sigmoidal curve results (pIC_{50} curve). The value of the abscissa corresponding to the half-maximal ordinate value of this curve is the IC_{50}, namely the molar concentration of antagonist that produces half-maximal inhibition of the defined agonist response. The same pIC_{50} curve would be obtained for any level of response.

The main reason for noting the patterns of antagonism produced by orthosteric antagonists with various rates of offset kinetics is to determine the correct method of estimating antagonist potency. As discussed previously, all antagonism can be estimated with a pIC_{50}, but there are circumstances where this empirical quantity differs from the correct pK_B (notably with simple competitive antagonists). The pA_2 can also be a useful estimate, but a full analysis of a range of concentrations of antagonists in a Schild analysis is needed to ensure identity of the pA_2 with the pK_B. Finally, a direct fit of curves for a simple competitive antagonist can yield an estimate of pK_B (Fig. 4.8). For true non-competitive (insurmountable) antagonism,

where the maximal response to the agonist is depressed, directly fitting experimental data requires a more explicit model than that available for simple competitive antagonism (i.e., equation 4.4). Specifically, a non-competitive model based on the Black–Leff operational model (see Chapter 3) can be used according to the equation shown below (Derivations and Proofs, Appendix B7):

$$\text{Response} = \frac{[A]^n\ \tau^n\ E_m}{[A]^n\ \tau^n + (([A] + K_A)([B]/K_B + 1))^n}$$

(4.6)

where K_A and τ are the affinity and efficacy of the agonist [A], E_m is the maximal response of

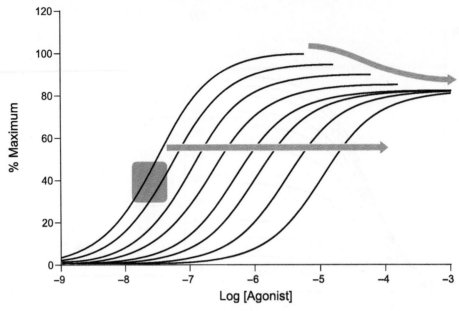

FIGURE 4.13   Antagonist hemi-equilibrium. Shown are the effects of increasing concentrations of a competitive antagonist in a system where there is insufficient time for complete re-equilibration between agonist, antagonist and receptors within the time-frame available to measure response to the agonist in the presence of the antagonist. This type of system is characterized by a depression of maximal response to a new steady-state level below that of the control curve but greater than zero. The antagonist potency can be estimated with Schild analysis or through estimation of the pA_2 (shaded rectangle).

the system, n is a slope fitting parameter and K_B is the equilibrium dissociation constant for the antagonist [B]. An example of the application of equation 4.6 to fitting data is shown in Fig. 4.14.

While the pattern of curves for antagonism observed *in vitro* is relevant to the quantification of antagonist potency, it is not as important in therapeutic use. Specifically, the production of competitive (surmountable) versus non-competitive antagonism can simply be a function of the way the antagonist is studied. The key factor here is the time allowed for the collection of agonist response in the presence of antagonist. If this time is short and insufficient for re-equilibration of agonist, antagonist and receptors to occur, then non-competitive antagonism will result. For example, a

truncated time for response collection is operative in measuring transient calcium release, a rapid process. Thus, many antagonists produce non-competitive antagonism in this type of assay. The very same antagonist may produce surmountable simple competitive antagonism (parallel shift to the right of curves with no depression of maximum) in another assay that allows a longer time for agonist, antagonist and receptor to re-equilibrate. Reporter assays, which incubate the ligands for 24 hours while gene expression takes place, are one such assay; thus, a given antagonist may be non-competitive in a calcium transient assay and surmountably competitive in a reporter assay (see Fig. 4.15).

The ultimate aim of these experiments is to utilize antagonists *in vivo* for therapeutic

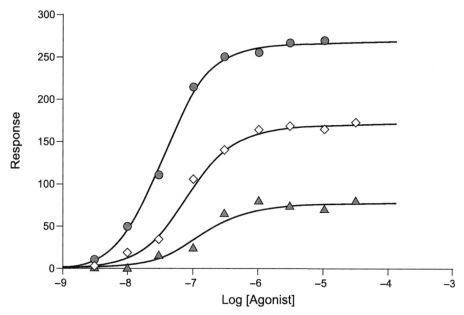

FIGURE 4.14 Dose–response curves obtained in the presence of increasing concentrations of a non-competitive antagonist fit to the model for non-competitive antagonism (equation 4.6).

advantage. Under these circumstances, the antagonist will enter a system already activated by agonist (much as in a pIC_{50} experiment) and produce a reduction in the basal response. Once the antagonist diffuses out of the receptor compartment (through whole body clearance; see Chapter 8), the basal response will be regained providing the steady-state function of the system has not otherwise changed. Since it would be postulated that most physiological systems will operate in a region sensitive to changes in the endogenous agonist concentration (lower region of the dose–response curve), the effects of antagonists on the high concentration end of the agonist dose–response curve probably are not relevant to whole body physiology. Figure 4.16 shows the *in vivo* effect of an antagonist on a basal agonist response. Figure 4.17 shows the *in vivo* responses of a simple competitive (surmountable) and a non-competitive (insurmountable) antagonist; it can be seen that the *in vivo* effects

are nearly identical. Therefore, the determination of competitive versus non-competitive mechanisms *in vitro* is important only from the point of view of using the correct model to measure the pK_B.

PARTIAL AND INVERSE AGONISTS

As discussed in Chapter 1, affinity and efficacy are generated by the same thermodynamic properties of the molecule, thus if a molecule has affinity for a given protein it is likely to have some kind of efficacy as well. Efficacy is the ability of the molecule to bind to and stabilize selective protein states, and to shift the equilibrium between protein states. Depending on the types of receptor states produced, this could result in a receptor with properties different from those of the unbound receptor. In terms of cell signaling, this difference could take the form of increased cellular

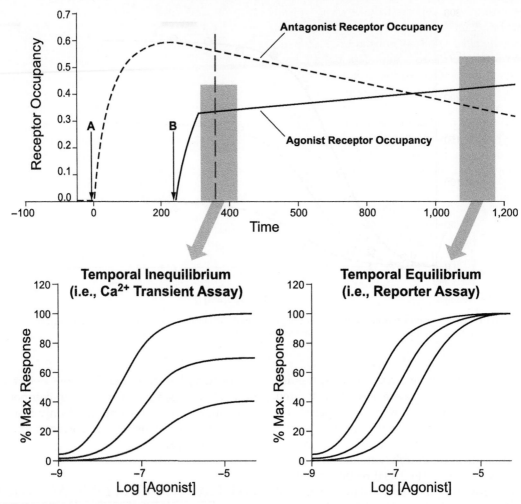

FIGURE 4.15   Effect of different time periods to measure agonist response (in the presence of a slowly dissociating orthosteric antagonist) shown in top panel. Panel on the left shows observed antagonism when the period for measurement of response is too short for complete re-equilibration (non-competitive antagonism is observed). Panel on the right shows the same system when sufficient time for the slowly dissociating antagonist is allowed for proper re-equilibration between agonist, antagonist and receptors. Under these circumstances, simple competitive antagonism is observed.

activity (positive agonism) or a decrease in elevated basal activity (inverse agonism). This latter condition occurs when the cell contains a critical mass of receptors already in an activated state; this could be because of mutation or high receptor expression. It is useful to think of the receptor population in any cell as a mixture of conformations (termed an "ensemble") with some preferred low energy conformations and others mediating cellular activity. Most systems are preset to the "inactive" conformations of receptors, thus the baseline cellular activity is low. A given antagonist could have preferred affinity for this "inactive" state or have a low affinity for an active state; these preferred affinities will shift the

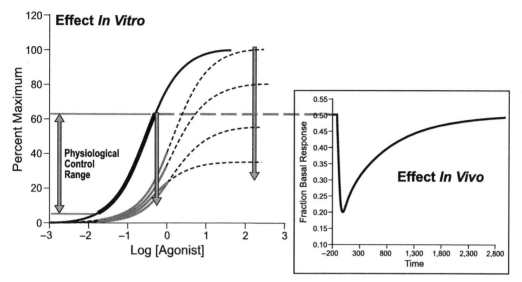

FIGURE 4.16   Effects of an antagonist *in vivo* where a level of basal activity is present. The dose–response curve to the endogenous agonist will be shifted to the right and/or depressed by the antagonist; the panel on the right shows the observed response *in vivo*. As the antagonist enters the receptor compartment and binds, the elevated basal response is depressed; as the antagonist washes out of the receptor compartment, the response returns.

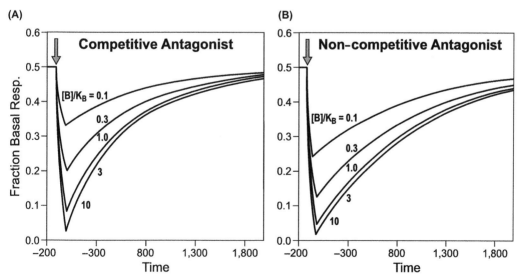

FIGURE 4.17   *In vivo* effects (see Fig. 4.16) of a competitive versus a non-competitive antagonist on endogenous elevated basal response.

equilibrium of the ensemble toward those preferred states and thus lead to observed cellular response.

First we will consider partial agonism. As shown in Fig. 4.18, a balance shows the predominant receptor species in a cell (inactive); an antagonist with positive efficacy will shift this toward activation and a response will be observed in systems sensitive enough to respond to the weak stimulus. Figure 4.19 shows the effect of a range of concentrations of partial agonist on the responses to a full agonist. The elevated baseline shows the intrinsic activation of the system by the partial agonist. The shift to the right of the full agonist dose—response curve shows how the partial agonist with lower efficacy occupies the receptor and blocks the effect of the more efficacious full agonist; thus a dual nature of partial agonists is revealed. They can function as agonists in sensitive systems, but can also function as antagonists of highly efficacious agonists. It is this dual nature of partial agonists (specifically with the β-adrenoceptor partial agonist dichloroisoproterenol) that intrigued James Black and his team at ICI and led them to discover and develop beta-blockers (see Box 4.4). The dextral displacement of the full agonist dose—response curves furnishes dose ratio values that can be used in Schild analysis to determine the pK_B of the partial agonist.

Another type of shift in protein conformational equilibrium leads to an opposite effect, namely inverse agonism. As noted, receptor proteins exist in collections of conformations and some of these spontaneously-formed active states may produce a cellular response (referred to as "constitutive activity"). One method of quantifying this effect is through an "allosteric constant" designated L, which is the spontaneous ratio of active receptor state (denoted $[R_a]$) and inactive receptor state ($[R_i]$) with the relation $L = [R_a]/[R_i]$. Thus a value of $L = 10^{-4}$ indicates that for every 10,000 receptors, one may be spontaneously in the active state at any one time. There are conditions, such as receptor mutation or receptor overexpression (e.g., cancer), where this ratio can lead to an elevated basal response. In the case of receptor overexpression, if a tumor cell expresses 1000 times more receptors on the cell surface, it can be seen that a receptor with $L = 10^{-4}$ may now produce an ambient level of 1000 active-state receptors, possibly enough to produce an elevated basal cellular response. Figure 4.20 shows such a system where the balance is now showing an elevated active-state receptor level. An antagonist with a preferred affinity for the active state will now reverse this elevated basal effect and produce a depression of cellular basal level of response. Figure 4.21 shows the effect of an inverse agonist on dose—response curves of a full agonist in a system demonstrating elevated constitutive activity. It should be noted that this same molecule will produce simple competitive

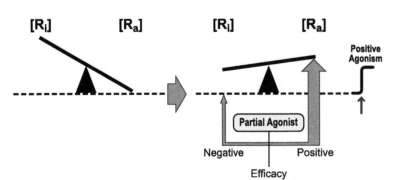

FIGURE 4.18 Receptor systems depicted as a balance between receptor active ($[R_a]$) and inactive ($[R_i]$) species. In the absence of agonist, the equilibrium for these systems lies far toward the $[R_i]$ state. A partial agonist, by virtue of having positive efficacy, shifts the balance toward a low level of active state receptor, thereby producing a low level of response.

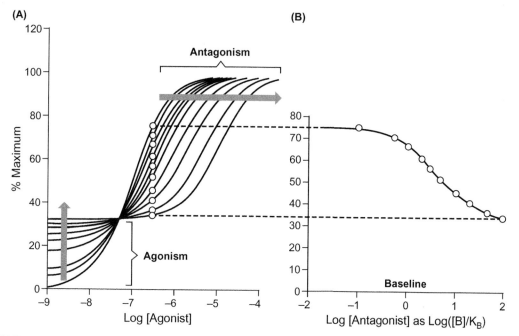

FIGURE 4.19 The effect of a partial agonist on the dose–response curve to an agonist. The partial agonist produces a direct response due to a low level of positive efficacy and it also shifts the dose–response curve to the agonist to the right. This competitive antagonist effect is the result of competition between the high efficacy agonist and lower efficacy partial agonist. The activity of the partial agonist as an antagonist can be determined with a pIC$_{50}$ curve (panel on the right); note how the direct effect of the partial agonist produces an elevated baseline for the pIC$_{50}$ curve. The shift to the right of the agonist dose–response curve can be used in Schild analysis to determine the pK$_B$.

blockade (i.e., effects such as those shown in Fig. 4.7) in cells with no constitutive activity. In this sense, the term inverse "agonist" is a misnomer, since these really are antagonists. However, since the reversal of elevated basal response can be seen as an overt change in cellular state, the term agonist has been used to describe these molecules. It can be seen from Fig. 4.21 that the constitutively elevated basal effect is depressed by the inverse agonist, but the dose–response curves to the full agonist are shifted to the right. Under these circumstances, this dextral displacement of the curves can be used for Schild analysis to calculate a pK$_B$ for antagonism. When discovered for 7TM receptors by Costa and Herz (see Box 4.5),[4] inverse agonism appeared to be an anomaly.

However, as more constitutively active systems became available for experimentation, it became clear that, as theoretically predicted, inverse agonism is the most prevalent form of antagonism and the depression of basal response becomes evident for these molecules only when the assay allows constitutively elevated activity to be observed. However, there are a sub-class of antagonists that presumably have similar affinities for [R$_a$] and [R$_i$] to the point that no change in basal effect is produced, even in constitutively active systems; this sub-class of antagonist is referred to as "neutral." It is not clear to what extent inverse agonism is a therapeutically relevant drug property, since most cell systems do not appear to be constitutively active. However, in

BOX 4.4

PARTIAL AGONISTS: DRUGS WITH TWO FACES

Partial agonists can cause activation of a quiescent system and antagonism of response in a system activated by a more efficacious agonist. This dichotomous behavior intrigued James Black (see Box 2.6) who noticed that dichloroisoproterenol (then known as Lilly 20522) blocked the effects of isoproterenol (see black tracing) in guinea pig trachea (redrawn from [5]) but otherwise was known to stimulate receptors like isoproterenol, but to a lesser extent. An example of this latter activity is shown in the dose–response curve for GTPγS activation, where 20522 produces a 30% maximal response to isoproterenol (redrawn from [6]). This apparently conflicting activity can be seen from the complete dose–response curves to an agonist in the absence and presence of a partial agonist. At lower values of basal activity, the stimulatory effect of the partial agonist is seen, whereas at higher response values the antagonism by the partial agonist dominates. Understanding this effect led Black and his team to develop the first beta-blockers.

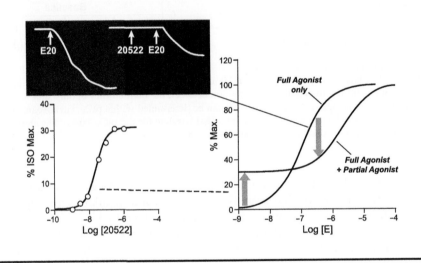

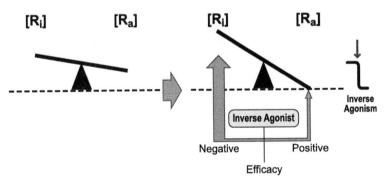

FIGURE 4.20 Receptor systems depicted as a balance between receptor active ($[R_a]$) and inactive ($[R_i]$) species. In a constitutively active receptor system, there is a low level of spontaneously formed active state receptor leading to an elevated basal response. An inverse agonist, by virtue of having negative efficacy, shifts the balance back toward a predominantly inactive receptor state, thereby reducing the endogenously elevated basal response.

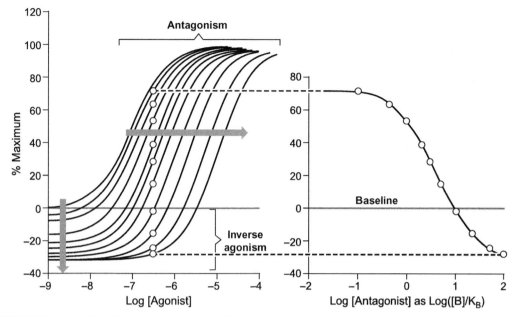

FIGURE 4.21 The effect of an inverse agonist on the dose–response curve to an agonist. If the receptor system is constitutively active then the baseline response will be spontaneously elevated. The inverse agonist produces a direct reversal of this elevated basal response due to a low level of negative efficacy; the inverse agonist also shifts the dose–response curve to the agonist to the right. The activity of the inverse agonist as an antagonist can be determined with a pIC_{50} curve (panel on the right); note how the direct effect of the inverse agonist produces a baseline for the pIC_{50} curve that is lower than the constitutively elevated baseline. The shift to the right of the agonist dose–response curve can be used in Schild analysis to determine the pK_B.

cases where they are (i.e., tumor growth), inverse agonists and neutral antagonists will have different properties.

If an antagonist molecule produces a receptor conformation of lower intrinsic ability to produce response than the spontaneously formed receptor active state ($[R_a]$), then an intriguing reversal of observed activity can occur. Specifically, such a molecule will produce positive activation of the receptor under normal circumstances but inverse agonism in cases where there is a high level of constitutive activity; such molecules are referred to as "protean agonists," named after the Greek mythological god Proteus who could change his shape at will (see Box 4.6).

ANTAGONIST EFFECTS *IN VIVO*

The interplay of the potency of a molecule as it induces antagonism and its intrinsic efficacy (either positive for partial agonists or negative for inverse agonists), and the ambient basal response of the system *in vivo* (either through presence of endogenous agonist or through constitutive activity) can combine to produce a complex array of observed effects *in vivo*. Figure 4.22 shows the possible outcomes of such molecules to *in vivo* systems of varying endogenous activation. In general, a rich array of potential therapeutic effects can be achieved through judicious choice of efficacy in candidate antagonist molecules.

BOX 4.5

THE DISCOVERY OF INVERSE AGONISM

Although negative agonism was noted for benzodiazepine receptors some years earlier, a paper by Costa and Herz[4] was the first to demonstrate inverse agonism for seven trans-membrane receptors. Working with opioid receptors in NG-108 cells, they showed that elevation of the basal response through changes in ionic media revealed a clear negative response to the peptide ICI174. Notably, the weakly positive response to MR2266 was not obvious until the basal response and assay sensitivity were elevated to a higher level with 150 mM KCl.

These data clearly showed how the observation of ligand efficacy depends on the setpoint of the assay. Increased sensitivity of the assay is optimal for demonstrating positive agonism (note MR226 in 150 NaCl) and increased basal response is optimal for showing inverse agonism (ICI174 in 150 KCl). Although considered an oddity when first published, inverse agonism is now seen to be a very common phenomenon by other researchers as they tested antagonists in constitutively active (elevated basal response) assays.

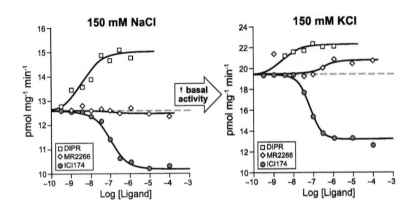

DESCRIPTIVE PHARMACOLOGY: IV

Chapters 1 to 3 discussed the effects of molecules that directly alter cellular function (agonists). Figure 4.23 shows two possible effects of molecules that, when added to a bimolecular system (reference agonist plus test molecule), can alter the effect of a reference agonist. Increases in response are discussed

further in Chapter 5. If response is diminished, then some form of antagonism is operative. As with agonism (see Chapter 2, Agonist Selectivity), the selectivity of the antagonism must be determined to differentiate effects from non-specific toxic or depressant activity. This can be done readily by demonstrating that no antagonism is produced to agonists of other receptors in the same preparation.

BOX 4.6

PROTEAN AGONISTS

Considering efficacy as the stabilization of a distinct ensemble of receptor conformations with the ability to induce a response, it should be noted that spontaneously formed receptor active states responsible for constitutive activity (elevated basal responses) also have an intrinsic efficacy (ability to induce response). In early formulations of receptor theory, it was assumed that agonists simply enrich levels of the naturally occurring active states(s), but subsequent research showed that many ligands can induce unique receptor conformations with varying levels of ability to produce cellular effect. If agonist stabilization produces an ensemble of lower efficacy to induce response than the naturally occurring receptor active state, then a phenomenon referred to as "protean" agonism can occur.[7] Named after the Greek mythological sea god Proteus who could change his shape at will, protean agonists such as dichloroisoproterenol are positive agonists in normal systems and inverse agonists in constitutively active systems. As shown by Chidiac and coworkers [8] in the graph below, DCI produces positive agonism in S9 cells. When membranes are produced from these cells that are spontaneously active and have an elevated basal response, DCI produces negative effects instead.

Isoproterenol → Dichloroisoproterenol

Figure 4.24 shows the possible array of responses to a purported antagonist and the resulting classifications of activity deduced from the observed response; these effects can be classified by the respective effects of the molecule on basal assay response and the maximal response of the assay to a full agonist. If the molecule blocks the effects of powerful full agonists, but also increases the basal response of an assay in its own right, then it is a partial agonist (assuming it produces surmountable antagonism of the full agonist effect). Under these circumstances, the dextral displacements of the full agonist dose–response curve can be used in Schild analysis to determine the pK_B. If the molecule decreases basal response, and especially if it can be determined that the basal response is constitutively elevated through spontaneous receptor activity, then it is likely that the molecule is an inverse agonist. Under these circumstances, the pK_B can be estimated through Schild analysis, as discussed in the section Orthosteric (Competitive and Non-Competitive) Antagonism in this chapter.

Finally, a molecule may produce no effect on basal response, but may otherwise antagonize the responses to a full agonist. If the maximal response to the full agonist is not affected, then this would be consistent with simple

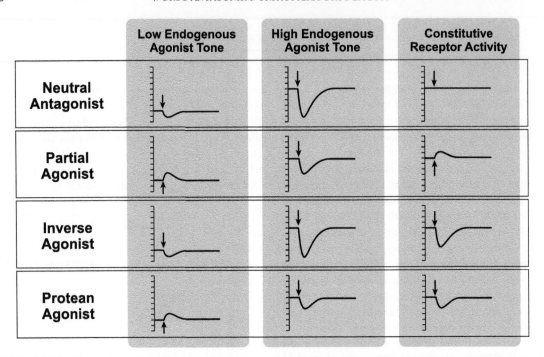

FIGURE 4.22   The *in vivo* effects of various antagonists. A neutral antagonist will block endogenous agonism but will have no effect on constitutively active agonism. A partial agonist may elevate response under conditions of low endogenous activation but block the effects of high endogenous agonism. A partial agonist will elevate response in a constitutively activated system if the level of constitutive activity is low. An inverse agonist will depress all response whether it is due to endogenous agonism or to constitutive receptor activity. A protean agonist will elevate response in conditions of low activation but will block the effects of both high endogenous agonism or constitutively elevated response.

competitive antagonism. The potency of the antagonist (as a pK_B) could then be estimated with Schild analysis. If an increase in the maximal response is produced by the molecule, then it is an allosteric modulator (see Chapter 5). If the molecule produces a depression of the maximal response, then a number of possibilities arise. The depression of maximum could be concentration-dependent and complete (i.e., a sufficiently high concentration of the antagonist will reduce the maximal response to zero). Under these circumstances, the effect could be a pseudo-irreversible orthosteric non-competitive blockade or an allosteric antagonism. Data can be fit to the

non-competitive model to yield a pK_B under these conditions. If the depression of maximal response reaches a limiting value and no further antagonism is produced by higher concentrations of antagonist, this suggests allosteric antagonism (see Chapter 5). If the maximal response is depressed to a limiting value greater than zero, but increasing concentrations of antagonist further shift the curve with a newly depressed maximum, this suggests a hemi-equilibrium state whereby a mixed pseudo-irreversible and competitive blockade is produced. Under these circumstances, Schild analysis can be used to estimate the pK_B.

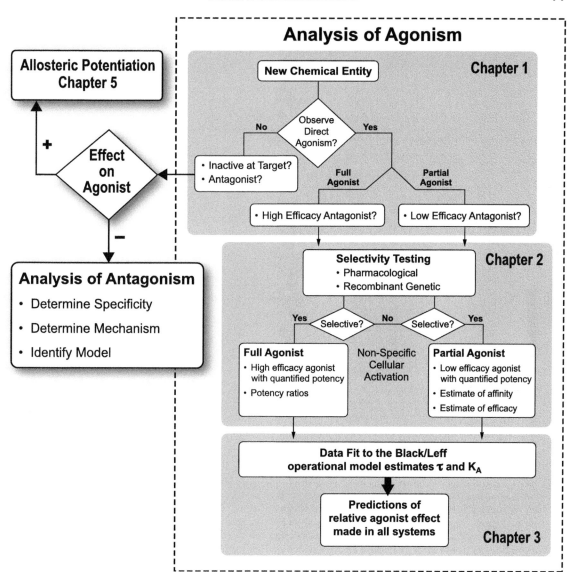

FIGURE 4.23 Descriptive pharmacology; schematic diagram of logic used to characterize drug effect. The characterization of agonism is shown in the area bounded by the dotted line (as described in Chapters 1 to 3). If no direct agonism is observed then the new chemical entity should be tested in a bi-molecular system consisting of the test compound and an endogenous agonist. If the level of endogenous agonism is elevated, then the test compound most likely is an allosteric positive modulator; these are discussed in the next chapter. If the endogenous agonism is depressed, then analysis continues to determine the mode of antagonism.

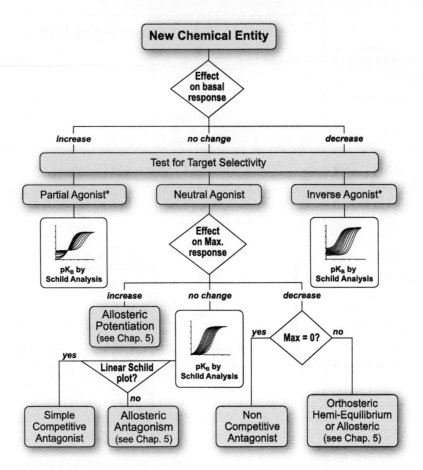

FIGURE 4.24   Schematic diagram depicting the logic used to determine the mode of action and potency of an antago-nist. It is assumed that relevant procedures are used to determine that the antagonism is specific for the target (see Fig. 4.2). The antagonist may elevate basal response, in which case it would be analyzed as a partial agonist. Similarly, if the molecule depressed basal activity it would be analyzed as an inverse agonist. If no effects on basal response are observed then the antagonism is classified in terms of the effects on the maximal response to the agonist. If no effect on maximal response is observed, then a Schild analysis is done to test for linearity of the Schild plot and adherence to the model of simple competitive antagonism. If the Schild plot is curvilinear, then further tests are done to determine possible allosteric antagonism (see Chapter 5). This is also the case if the antagonist produces an increased maximal response to the agonist. If the maximal response to the agonist is depressed, then the nature of this depression is explored further. Specifically, the degree to which maximal response is depressed is examined; if the maximal response can be completely depressed to baseline, then an orthosteric non-competitive antagonism is suggested (although it is still possible that a high level of negative co-operativity in a negative allosteric modulator could also cause this; see Chapter 5). If the antago-nism reaches a new steady-state beyond which no further antagonism occurs, then a negative allosterism is suggested (see Chapter 5). If the maximal response is depressed to a new steady-state but further dextral displacement of the curve occurs, then an orthosteric hemi-equilibrium is suggested.

SUMMARY

- There are two possible modes of action of antagonism; orthosteric blockade (occlusion of the agonist binding site) and allosteric modulation.
- Antagonism is characterized by the quantity of antagonist bound (*potency*), the location of the binding relative to the binding of the natural agonist (*mechanism*) and the persistence of antagonist binding (*antagonist kinetics*).
- The relative rates of dissociation of the antagonist from the receptor, the rate of association of the agonist with the receptor and the length of time available to achieve equilibrium determine whether surmountable or insurmountable blockade will be observed.
- Simple competitive blockade occurs when there is sufficient time to achieve equilibrium; it is characterized by parallel shifts to the right of agonist curves with no depression of maximum.
- Competitive antagonism is quantified with a pK_B value determined through Schild analysis.
- If the rate of dissociation of the antagonist is slow it can effectively irreversibly block a portion of the receptor population and a depression of the maximal response to the agonist can result.
- A mixture of the above effects can occur whereby a portion of the receptors are essentially irreversibly blocked; this is referred to as hemi-equilibrium and results in partially depressed maxima with shifts to the right of the curve(s).
- Estimates of antagonist potency can be obtained for all modes of antagonism through a pA_2 value and/or a pIC_{50} of antagonism of a fixed agonist effect.
- Antagonists can produce low levels of positive response (partial agonists) or depression of basal responses elevated by constitutive receptor activity (inverse agonists).
- Surmountable versus insurmountable antagonism has little relevance to antagonism *in vivo* since reduction in basal response is the main effect observed in these systems.

QUESTIONS

4.1 A given orthosteric antagonist produces a shift to the right of the agonist dose−response curve with no depression of maximum, and a further shift with a depression of maximum at higher doses. What might be happening?

4.2 A rapid estimate of the potency of an antagonist of unknown potency is required. What would be a good method of doing this?

4.3 A given antagonist produces surmountable simple competitive blockade in one type of assay and a depression of agonist maximal response in another. The chemist is worried that there is a problem in the testing; why should this not be a concern?

4.4 A pIC_{50} is measured for an antagonist and surprisingly, the maximal response for antagonism falls well below basal response of the assay. What could be happening and what does this say about the antagonist in question?

References

[1] J.H. Gaddum, The quantitative effects of antagonistic drugs, J. Physiol. Lond. 89 (1937) 7P−9P.

[2] O. Arunlakshana, H.O. Schild, Some quantitative uses of drug antagonists, Br. J. Pharmacol. 14 (1959) 48−58.

[3] P. Leff, I.G. Dougall, Further concerns over Cheng−Prusoff analysis, Trends Pharmacol. Sci. 14 (1993) 110−112.

[4] T. Costa, A. Herz, Antagonists with negative intrinsic activity at δ-opioid receptors coupled to GTP-binding proteins, Proc. Natl. Acad. Sci. USA 86 (1989) 7321−7325.

[5] C.E. Powell, I.H. Slater, Blocking of inhibtory adrenergic receptors by a dichloro analog of isoproterenol, J. Pharmacol. Exp. Ther. 122 (1958) 480−488.

[6] C. Ambrosio, P. Molinari, F. Fanelli, Y. Chuman, M. Sbraccia, O. Ugur, et al., Different structural requirements for the constitutive and agonist-induced activities for the β2-adrenergic receptor, J. Biol. Chem. 280 (2005) 23464−23474.

[7] T.P. Kenakin, Protean agonists: Keys to receptor active state? Ann. New York Acad. Sci. 812 (1997) 116−125.

[8] P. Chidiac, T.E. Hebert, M. Valiquette, M. Dennis, M. Bouvier, Inverse agonist activity of β-adrenergic antagonists, Mol. Pharmacol. 45 (1994) 490−499.

5

Allosteric Drug Effects

By the end of this chapter the reader will know the characteristic properties of allosteric molecules and how they interact with proteins. In addition, the reader will know strategies for identifying allosterism and the reasons why this is relevant to drug discovery. Specifically, these involve the unique therapeutic properties of allosteric modulators. Finally, the reader will learn how to use pharmacologic tools to quantify allosteric behavior of molecules for use in studies aimed at optimization of allosteric activity.

INTRODUCTION

Conventional concepts about drug discovery center on the assumption that a drug must have an affinity for a naturally physiologically relevant site on a biological target. For instance, antimuscarinic antagonists such as scopolamine are targeted toward the acetylcholine binding site on the acetylcholine receptor. Similarly, many kinase inhibitors are targeted toward the natural ATP binding site of kinases. These systems, as discussed in Chapter 4, can be thought of as "orthosteric" in nature since steric hindrance may play an important role in the mechanism of action. Allosteric molecules can bind to virtually any site on the target protein and affect its activity; this greatly expands the possible therapeutic opportunities for a given target. This may be an extremely important approach, as it is known that if a molecule is bound to the protein at any site the conformational movement of that protein may be affected (*vide infra*). These effects are allosteric and have become a very important part of new drug discovery.

NEW TERMINOLOGY

The following new terms will be introduced in this chapter:

- α: Denoted within the standard model for functional allosterism quantifying the effect of an allosteric modulator on the affinity of a protein for another molecule.
- β: Denoted within the standard model for functional allosterism quantifying the effect of an allosteric modulator on the efficacy of an agonist binding to a receptor protein.
- **Co-operativity**: The effective interaction between the two co-binding allosteric molecules on the protein, i.e., the effect of one of the ligands on the affinity and efficacy of the other.
- **Ensemble**: A collection of protein conformations visualized as a snapshot in time in a dynamic system whereby the protein spontaneously samples an enormously large library of conformations.
- **Modulator (allosteric)**: A molecule that co-binds with another on a protein to affect the behavior of the protein toward the cell and the co-binding ligand.
- **Negative allosteric modulator (NAM)**: An allosteric modulator that antagonizes agonist activation of a receptor, i.e., reduces the affinity and/or the efficacy of an agonist for a receptor (an allosteric antagonist).
- **Positive allosteric modulator (PAM)**: An allosteric modulator that promotes agonist activation of a receptor, i.e., increases the affinity and/or the efficacy of an agonist for a receptor.
- **Probe dependence**: Variation of activity of an allosteric modulator as it modifies the protein interaction with various probes (radioligands, agonists).

PROTEIN ALLOSTERISM

Allosteric interactions on proteins such as receptors and ion channels occur through the binding of a molecule onto the protein to affect its free energy of conformation. This subsequently affects the behavior of the protein toward the cell, other proteins and ligands. The change in behavior occurs through a change in conformation of the protein. The energy of the protein changes upon ligand binding no matter how relatively small the molecule is in relation to the protein. There are a number of proposed mechanisms for protein allostery, ranging from the existence of low energy pathways between binding sites (allosteric "hot wires") to the stabilization of global protein conformations. A major milestone in the consideration of protein behavior was given by Koshland[1] who described how structured enzymes (modeled by the historical "lock-and-key" model of rigid proteins) accommodated substrates through movement of amino acid residues ("induced fit;" see Box 5.1). For receptors, this induced fit model is less applicable than the conformational selection model discussed in Chapter 2 (see Fig 2.6 and Box 2.5) describing the stabilization of global protein conformations through ligand binding. Receptors and other protein drug targets are complex macromolecules that exist in a multitude of tertiary interconvertable conformations (shapes). At any one instant, a collection of protein molecules will have a selection of different conformations of similar free energy; these collections are called ensembles. As discussed in Chapter 2, the binding of a ligand initiates a process of conformational selection within the ensemble where the ligand preferentially binds to the conformations for which it has the highest affinity at the expense of others. If the enriched protein species mediates cellular response then the ligand is an agonist. In this chapter, ligands that produce a conformational

BOX 5.1

KOSHLAND AND INDUCED FIT INTO PROTEINS

In 1894, Emil Fischer accounted for the extraordinary specificity of enzyme–substrate interactions with a description of a strict geometric complementarity; this idea became famous as a "lock-and-key" hypothesis for recognition between molecules and proteins. While this explained enzyme recognition of substrates, it did not account for the stabilization of a new state of the enzyme referred to as the "transition state" needed to induce enzyme catalysis. Daniel Koshland, working at the University of California, Berkely, recognized that proteins are flexible structures and hypothesized that they accommodate the substrate by molding their shape around it; the substrate may also change its shape to optimize a conformation ideal for catalysis. This idea, referred to as "induced fit," overturned a 100-year-old view of how enzymes function and paved the way for allosteric theories of enzyme and receptor mechanisms.

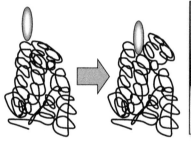 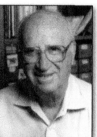

Daniel Koshland
(1920-2007)

change to affect the behavior of the protein toward other molecules will be considered; these molecules are referred to as **allosteric modulators**.

Protein allostery describes the process of *co-operativity* between binding sites, i.e., the binding of a molecule at one site on the protein alters the subsequent interaction of the protein with other molecules binding at other sites. One of the earliest models of allosterism in proteins, termed the Monod–Wyman–Changeux model,[2] describes the binding of molecules to proteins made up of multiple subunits, whereby the binding of a molecule to one subunit alters the subsequent binding of molecules to other subunits. Figure 5.1 shows the binding of a molecule to a single subunit and to a trimeric protein consisting of three subunits where the binding of each promotes the binding of the next (positive co-operativity). This produces a steep curve with a slope greater than unity for a Hill coefficient. Such binding behavior can be advantageous in physiology; for example, tetrameric co-operativity of oxygen binding to hemoglobin optimizes the delivery of oxygen to tissues (see Box 5.2).

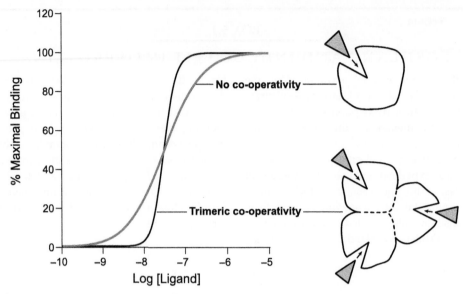

FIGURE 5.1 Dose–response curve for the binding of a ligand to a single subunit protein according to the Langmuir isotherm (equation 2.1, curve in gray marked "no co-operativity") and to a protein made up of three identical co-operatively linked subunits (black curve labeled "trimeric co-operativity"). For the trimer the binding of the ligand to one subunit promotes the binding to the second and the third, causing the binding curve to be steeper than that for a monomer.

Allosteric ligands bind to their own site on the protein. This opens the possibility of also binding the endogenous ligand as a co-binding ligand. This geographical distinction between binding sites was one of the first features of allosterism to be discovered. Specifically, the modification of biosynthetic enzyme activity, through binding of a structurally unrelated downstream product of biosynthetic pathways (as in the case of the biosynthesis of isoleucine [3]), was one of the first indications that proteins such as enzymes can bind molecules at multiple sites to modify their activity (Fig. 5.2). The binding of molecules to separate sites leads to a permissive system (whereby the action of one of the ligands may not necessarily preclude the action of another); this can facilitate an interaction between the endogenous ligand and the modulator. It also means that the behavior of the modulator-bound protein can vary for different co-binding ligands. This is one of the most important features of allostery, namely *probe dependence*. If the endogenous ligand is thought of as a probe of receptor function, then a given allosteric modulator can have *different* effects on different probes. The second important feature of allostery is *saturation of effect*. Unlike competitive mechanisms where effects can continue as long as different quantities of the interactants are added to the system, allosteric effects cease when the allosteric site on the protein is saturated. These properties of probe dependence and saturation of effect will surface repeatedly throughout this chapter as the specific properties of allosteric modulators are discussed.

TYPES OF ALLOSTERIC MODULATORS

There are no *a priori* rules for how a given allosteric modulator will affect the action of

BOX 5.2

ALLOSTERY AT WORK: CO-OPERATIVE BINDING OF OXYGEN TO HEMOGLOBIN

Hemoglobin is a tetrameric protein that binds and transports four oxygen molecules per unit and then releases them to myoglobin. The binding of oxygen to hemoglobin is allosterically co-operative, in that the binding of each oxygen molecule facilitates the binding of the next. As shown on the curve to the right, this produces a steep binding curve ideal for oxygen binding, transport and release. It can be seen from these curves that oxygen readily binds to hemoglobin at the high pO_2 values in the lung (100 torr). However, in tissues with lower oxygen levels (pO_2 20–40 torr) the co-operative binding of oxygen to hemoglobin causes the oxygen binding to drop off sharply. This allows hemoglobin to release the oxygen to myoglobin. It can be seen that the non-co-operative binding of oxygen to myoglobin causes it to be more tightly bound in this region of oxygen tension (20–40 torr).

The co-operative binding of oxygen is caused by the interaction of the four subunits of hemoglobin, whereby the binding of an oxygen molecule to one subunit increases the affinity of the remaining subunits for oxygen.

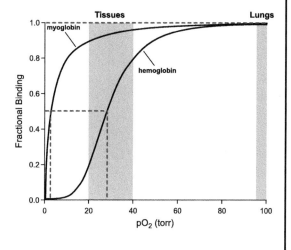

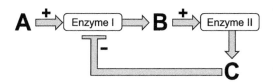

FIGURE 5.2 Negative feedback inhibition by the product of an enzyme cascade. The product of enzyme II (compound C) is structurally unrelated to substrate A, yet inhibits enzyme I through an allosteric site. This system is optimal for control of output since the overall product then controls the initial rate of the reaction cascade.

receptor probes. If the responsiveness of the receptor is reduced to a given probe, then the molecule is an *allosteric antagonist* (see Fig. 5.3). It should be noted that the principle of probe dependence dictates that different probes may be affected in different ways. Thus, an allosteric antagonist may block some agonists but not others (Fig. 5.3). The pattern of antagonism can vary from being surmountable to

being insurmountable. A discerning feature of allosteric antagonists is that they can produce a maximal asymptotic effect (when the allosteric site is fully occupied); the maximal effect they have on a receptor system is determined by co-operativity factors (*vide infra*). This fact can be used to differentiate allosteric antagonism from orthosteric antagonism. For example, a given surmountable allosteric effect may produce

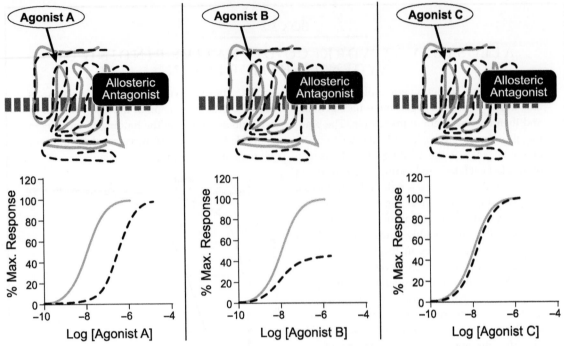

FIGURE 5.3 Probe dependence of an allosteric antagonist for three agonists A, B and C. The modulator produces surmountable antagonism of responses to agonist A, a non-competitive antagonism of responses to B and no effect at all on responses to agonist C. Such behavior is characteristic of allestoric modulators.

shifts to the right of the agonist dose–response curve that come to a maximal value (see Fig. 5.4A). Under these circumstances, Schild analysis in such a system produces a distinct curvature of the Schild plot (Fig. 5.4B). The use of this concept to identify allosterism is discussed later in this chapter. Some allosteric modulators can also increase the responsiveness of protein targets; these are referred to as positive allosteric modulators (PAMs) (see Fig. 5.5). The effects of PAMS are also subject to probe dependence.

An allosteric effect in a protein basically can change the complete behavior of that protein and the way it interacts with other molecules. Thus, in the case of a receptor and endogenous agonists, an allosteric modulator can change

the affinity of the agonist, the efficacy of the agonist, or both, and these changes need not be in the same direction. Figure 5.6A shows the effect of an allosteric modulator on the affinity of full and partial agonists; an increased affinity causes a shift to the left of the dose–response curve, and a decreased affinity causes a shift to the right. Figure 5.6B shows the effect of allosteric changes in the efficacy of full and partial agonists. In this case, an increased efficacy will shift the curve to a full agonist to the left, whereas for a partial agonist it will produce an increase in the maximal response. Similarly, a decreased efficacy can shift the dose–response curve to a full agonist with a high receptor reserve to the right or, in cases of smaller receptor reserves,

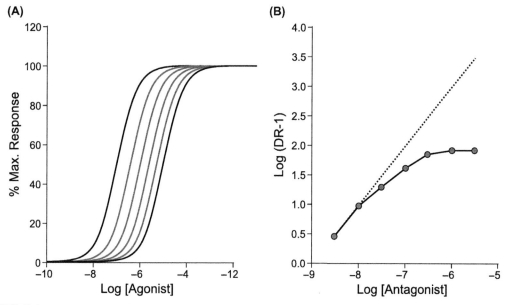

(A)

(B)

FIGURE 5.4 Surmountable allosteric antagonism. Panel A shows the limited antagonism produced by an allosteric antagonist; the limit of antagonism is reached when the concentration of modulator fully saturates the allosteric binding site. This limit of dextral displacement of the dose–response curves is reflected in a downward curvature in the Schild regression (Panel B); such curvilinear Schild regressions are characteristic of surmountable allosteric antagonists.

depress the maximal response. For a partial agonist, which by definition has no receptor reserve, a decrease in efficacy will depress the maximal response (see Fig. 5.6B). At this point it is worth considering how these properties of allosteric modulators can lead to unique drug behaviors therapeutically.

UNIQUE EFFECTS OF ALLOSTERIC MODULATORS

To discuss the unique effects of allosteric modulators it is first useful to consider orthosteric antagonists. These are molecules that preclude access of other molecules, such as agonists, to the receptor; these types of preemptive systems lead to the same maximal result, namely an inactivated (or in the case of partial agonists, a partially activated) receptor

to all agonism. In contrast, allosteric molecules are permissive in that they potentially allow interaction of the protein with other molecules; the result of an allosterically modulated system can be different for different agonists. This and the property of saturation of effect cause allosteric modulators to have a unique range of activities. These are:

1. **The potential to alter the interaction of very large proteins**. A hallmark of large protein–protein effects is that they probably involve multiple areas of interaction. Under these conditions an orthosteric ligand (one that alters only a single region of the protein) would be predicted to be minimally effective. However, an allosteric ligand that stabilizes a new global conformation of the protein (see Fig. 5.7) has the potential to alter the position of

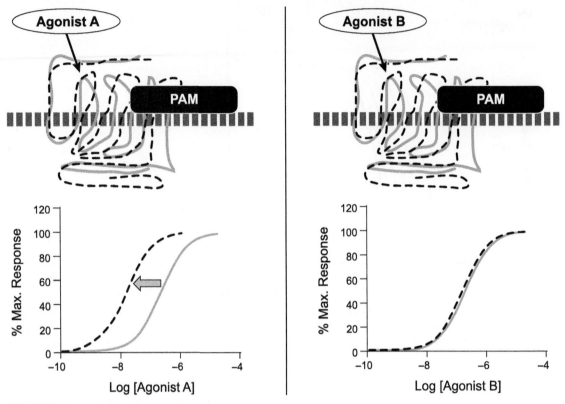

FIGURE 5.5 Probe dependence of a positive allosteric modulator (PAM) for two agonists A and B. While the modulator potentiates responses to agonist A, no effect is seen on agonist B. As with allosteric antagonism, such behavior is characteristic of allosteric modulators.

numerous areas of the protein, and thereby affect large protein–protein interactions. An example of this type of effect is the blockade of the interaction of the chemokine CCR5 receptor and the HIV-1 virus coat protein gp120 (both large proteins) by the allosteric ligand aplaviroc (1/200 the size of the proteins) to prevent HIV-1 infection.[4]

2. **The potential to modulate but not completely activate and/or inhibit receptor function.** The saturation of allosteric effect upon complete occupancy of the allosteric site allows allosteric modulators to produce limited effects on target proteins. For example, an allosteric antagonist may

produce only a maximal ten-fold decrease in the affinity of the receptor for a given agonist (Fig. 5.8A). As can be seen from Fig. 5.8A, a pIC_{50} plot (see Chapter 4) under these conditions yields a curve that does not reach the baseline. This is a hallmark of allosteric antagonist modulators that have limited maximal effects on receptors. The same net effect can be seen with allosteric antagonists that reduce the efficacy of receptor agonists (see Fig. 5.8B). Thus, it can be seen that, unlike an orthosteric antagonist, an allosteric antagonist modulator can reduce the responsiveness of a target without completely blocking its

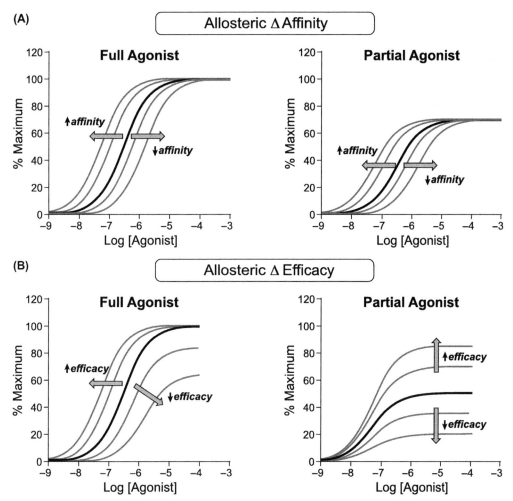

FIGURE 5.6 The various possible effects of an allosteric modulator on the response to an agonist. Panel A: Changes in the affinity of the receptor for both full and partial agonists result in shifts along the concentration axis of the dose−response curves (to the left for increased affinity and to the right for decreased affinity). Panel B: Effects of modulator-induced increases or decreases in agonist efficacy differ for full and partial agonists. Since the system cannot show further increased maximal responses to a full agonist, modulator-induced increased efficacy results in shifts to the left of the dose−response curve to a full agonist. For a partial agonist, the maximal response will increase. For decreases in efficacy, the maximal response to a partial agonist will decrease. This may also occur for a full agonist, although this will depend on the magnitude of the receptor reserve for the full agonist (i.e., see Fig. 4.11). Therefore, if there is high receptor reserve for the full agonist, a modulator-induced decrease in efficacy may result in a shift to the right of the dose−response curve with little depression of maximum. If the receptor reserve is small, then a modulator-induced decrease in efficacy will result in a depression of the maximal response.

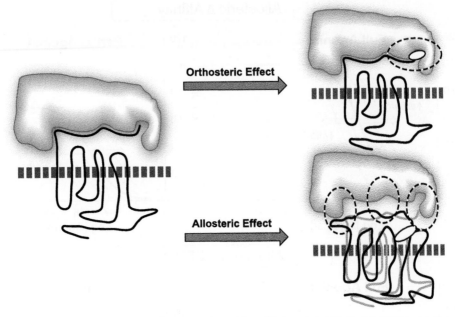

FIGURE 5.7 Disruption of the interaction of two proteins with multiple points of interaction. Top panel shows how an orthosteric molecule may interfere with protein–protein interaction at the site of binding. Bottom panel shows how stabilization of different global protein conformation can alter numerous regions of the protein to correspondingly affect numerous regions of interaction between the proteins.

function. Another feature of saturability is that it can disassociate the length of time of target blockade from the degree of blockade, i.e., high doses of a limited allosteric antagonist can allow a strategy whereby the production of a pool of drug gives a long lasting effect without overdose (see Box 5.3).

3. **Preservation of physiological patterns**. While direct agonism produces blanket activation of systems, positive allosteric modulators (PAMs) potentiate the existing responses in proportion to the natural physiological tone. This may be important in regions such as the brain, where failing complex patterns of neurological signaling may need to be augmented (as in diseases such as Alzheimer's).

4. **Reduction in side-effects**. A PAM produces no direct effect, but rather has an action only when the system is active through the presence of the natural agonist. Under these conditions, it would be expected that a lower side-effect profile for the PAM would be observed.

5. **Can produce texture in antagonism**. While orthosteric antagonists all produce a common end product upon saturation of binding (namely an inoperative biological target), allosteric antagonists produce antagonism through alterations of protein conformation, and these need not be identical. Under these circumstances, different allosteric modulators could produce pharmacological blockade through production of different protein conformations. This may be of importance in diseases such as AIDs where it is expected that HIV-1 viral mutation will

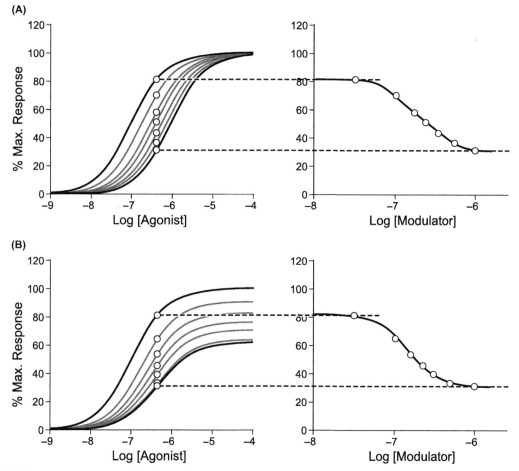

FIGURE 5.8 pIC_{50} curves for allosteric antagonists that produce limited maximal blockade of functional effects. (A) The pIC_{50} curve for a surmountable allosteric antagonist that produces a limited maximal shift to the right of the agonist dose–response curve may have a maximal value of inhibition that is above the baseline value of no agonism. (B) The same effect can occur with a non-competitive allosteric modulator that produces a limited maximal blockade.

eventually lead to tolerance to an HIV-1 entry inhibitor as the virus mutates to a form that can utilize the allosterically modified receptor. Therapy with a different allosteric modulator (one that produces a different conformation) could overcome this viral resistance.

6. **Can have separate effects on agonist affinity and efficacy**. There is no *a priori* rule to dictate that allosteric changes need

be in the same vectorial direction (antagonism or potentiation). Thus, it is possible to have an allosteric modulator that changes agonist affinity in one direction and efficacy in another (see Fig. 5.9). One particular combination of these activities can be useful, namely an allosteric antagonist modulator that increases agonist affinity but decreases agonist efficacy. The outcome of this combination is an

BOX 5.3

HIGH TARGET COVERAGE WITHOUT OVERDOSE

The fact that allosteric effects are saturable (the effect stops when the allosteric site is fully occupied) can lead to a maximal asymptote for antagonism. This can, in turn, lead to a dissociation of the intensity effect and duration of action. Specifically, to achieve a long-lasting effect, high doses of an antagonist must be used. With an orthosteric antagonist, this will, in turn, produce a large maximal effect which may lead to toxic interactions. In contrast, an allosteric antagonist achieves a self-limiting maximal effect. Increasing the dosage of such a molecule will not produce overdose, but will rather only prolong the effect *in vivo*.

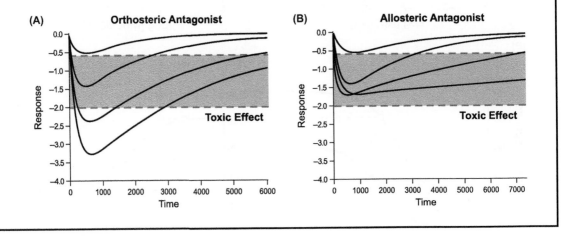

antagonist that becomes more potent with higher agonist concentrations, i.e., the antagonist develops use dependence (see Box 5.4).

7. **Allosteric modulators exercise "probe dependence."** Allosterism involves a change in the shape of the protein, and it is quite possible that a given change in shape could be catastrophic to the activity of one probe (i.e., agonist) but have no effect at all on another, especially if those probes bind to different regions of the protein. This has ramifications for the therapeutic application and also for the mode of discovery of allosteric modulators. In terms of the impact of probe dependence on therapeutic

application of allosteric modulators, the possibility exists that a given modulator could block or potentiate the endogenous agonist and have no effect on other receptor probes. For example, the CCR5 chemokine receptor mediates HIV-1 entry, leading to infection. However, activation of the CCR5 receptor by natural chemokines also offers protection against progression to AIDS after infection. Therefore, an ideal HIV-1 entry inhibitor would block the utilization of CCR5 by HIV-1 but otherwise allow normal chemokine function for this receptor; this is possible with allosteric modulators. In support of this idea, varying relative activities of allosteric modulators for HIV-1

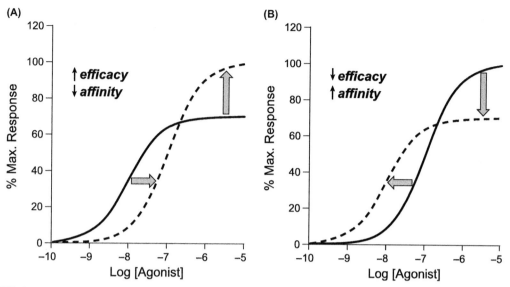

FIGURE 5.9 Effects of allosteric modulators that have opposite effects on agonist affinity and efficacy. (A) The alloste-ric ligand reduces agonist affinity and increases efficacy of a partial agonist; this will shift the dose–response curve to the right but increase maximal response. (B) A modulator that increases the affinity of the agonist but decreases the efficacy may shift the dose–response curve to the left (although the two effects may cancel to make this shift minimal) and will decrease the maximal response.

entry versus chemokine function have been noted experimentally.[5] In terms of how allosteric modulators are discovered and developed, this same probe dependence dictates that the endogenous ligand (i.e., the one that is targeted therapeutically) should be used in the screening and discovery process. For example, a PAM would be of use in augmenting a failing cholinergic neuronal transmission in Alzheimer's disease. However, the natural agonist (acetylcholine) is chemically unsuitable for use in a drug discovery screen and subsequent experiments. Under these circumstances, stable analogs, namely carbachol and/or pilocarpine, are often used in the screening process. However, probe dependence predicts that the activity of allosteric ligands could be very different for natural versus synthetic ligands. For example, it has been observed that PAMs

such as LY2033298 cause agonist-dependent differential potentiation of different agonists such as acetylcholine and oxotremorine.[6] This is also relevant to PAMs for targets with multiple natural agonists. For example, the antidiabetic PAM NOVO2 produces a five-fold potentiation of one of the natural agonists for the GLP-1 receptor GLP-1(7-36) NH_2, but a 25-fold potentiation of oxyntomodulin, another natural agonist for this receptor.[7] These data suggest that all agonists for a given receptor need to be tested when studying the effects of allosteric modulators.

DETECTING ALLOSTERISM

If a ligand potentiates endogenous signaling through binding to a target protein, it clearly is an allosteric ligand, i.e., potentiation would

BOX 5.4

USE DEPENDENCE FOR ALLOSTERIC ANTAGONISTS

An allosteric antagonist stabilizes a unique receptor protein conformation, and this can lead to differences in agonist affinity and/or efficacy. A modulator that increases the affinity of the agonist and decreases its efficacy can become more potent as the physiological system it is designed to block is driven to higher levels of activity; a "use dependence." This is due to the reciprocal nature of allosteric energy transfer. Thus, just as the modulator increases the affinity of the agonist, so too will the agonist increase the affinity of the allosteric antagonist. Therefore, the affinity of the antagonist will increase as the agonist concentration increases. Since the presence of the antagonist on the receptor precludes activation by the agonist (the modulator decreases agonist efficacy), the antagonism will increase as the concentration of agonist increases. Thus, the IC_{50} for blockade of a given level of response will decrease for the blockade of a higher level of response (i.e., see graph where the IC_{50} at 90% is $<IC_{50}$ at 50%). This type of activity is seen of the NMDA blocker ifenprodil[9] and the cannabinoid CB1 receptor blocker Org27569.[10]

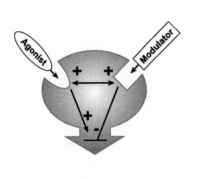
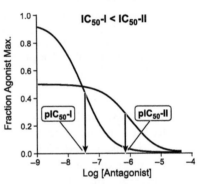

occur only through the co-binding of endogenous agonist and modulator. However, for antagonists, it may not be immediately clear whether the effect is orthosteric or allosteric, since both mechanisms can produce surmountable or insurmountable blockade. There are two strategies that can be used to detect allosteric antagonism. The first is through elevation of the range of concentrations tested; this approach can be used to uncover saturation of effect (i.e., detect curvature in Schild regressions to observe a maximal plateau in antagonist effect). Figure 5.10A shows the effect of a surmountable allosteric antagonist and how the shifts to the right of the dose—response curves differ from those of an equipotent orthosteric simple competitive antagonist. As shown in Fig. 5.4B, the saturation in maximal shift to the right of the curve results in a curvilinear Schild regression. Figure 5.10B shows a comparable saturation of effect for a non-competitive (insurmountable) allosteric antagonist. In this case, an orthosteric antagonist will reduce the agonist response to

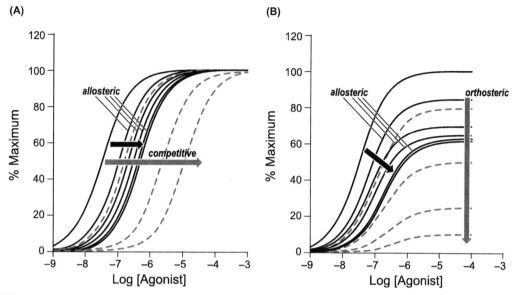

FIGURE 5.10 Saturation of allosteric effect. An allosteric antagonist modulator will have a limited maximal antago-nism (although this may be quite large for some modulators) which may become evident when a wide range of con-centrations of modulator are tested. (A) Whereas a simple competitive orthosteric antagonist will produce theoretically limitless shifts to the right of the agonist dose–response curve (broken gray lines), an allosteric modula-tor effect will cease when the allosteric site is saturated (black line curves). (B) Similarly, high concentrations of an orthosteric non-competitive antagonist will depress the maximal response to an agonist to baseline values (broken gray lines), whereas an allosteric non-competitive antagonist may block to a maximal effect above baseline (black line curves).

baseline (zero response to the agonist) when given in a suitably high concentration, whereas an allosteric antagonist may not. The other approach to detecting allosterism is through probe dependence; testing as many agonists as possible may uncover agonist-related differ-ences in effect.

To definitively confirm allosteric effect, changes in the kinetics of interaction of the protein target with agonists and/or other probes (i.e., radioligands) must be determined, since such changes can only be produced by allosteric ligands. The basis for this mechanism is the chemical nature of the association (k_1) and dissociation (k_2) kinetics of ligands for protein receptors; both of these mechanisms depend on the tertiary conformation of the protein. Specifically, both k_1 and k_2 are unique for every protein conformation/ligand pairing;

therefore, if a ligand produces a change in either k_1 or k_2 for another ligand, this can only occur through a change in the conformation of the protein. If an allosteric ligand produces potentiation of effect, then the K_{eq} either for binding or effect will decrease, i.e., the potency of the agonist will increase. Since K_{eq} is k_2/k_1 (see Chapter 2), then potentiation (decrease in K_{eq}) can occur either through a decrease in k_2 (decrease in rate of dissociation) or an increase in k_1 (increase in rate of association), or some combination of these. The rate of dissociation of an agonist can be measured by viewing the decay of response of an agonist after washing and addition of a high concentration of antago-nist. The antagonist is used to prevent rebind-ing of the agonist during the washout stage; under these circumstances, the decay of response reflects the k_2. Most PAM effects

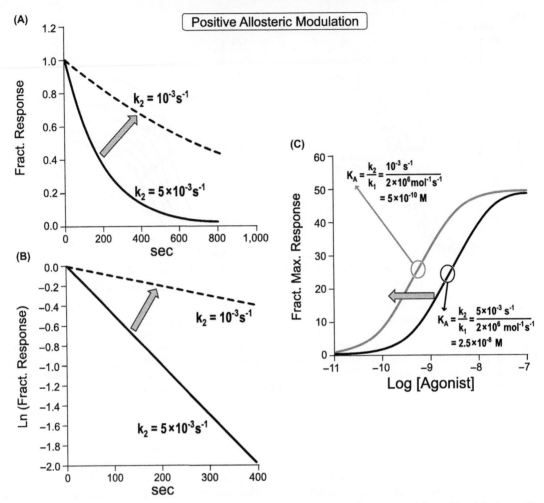

FIGURE 5.11   Alteration of kinetics of receptor dissociation by a positive allosteric modulator. Panel A shows the off-set of receptor response to an agonist in the presence of a high concentration of a competitive antagonist; this reversal of response reflects the rate of dissociation of the agonist from the receptor (k_2). The solid line represents the system in the absence of the allosteric modulator; the dotted line shows the decrease in the offset rate (and subsequent decrease in the rate of dissociation) in the presence of the PAM. It can be seen that the k_2 value decreases by a factor of 5. Panel B shows the same plot on a log ordinate scale (fractional response expressed as the natural logarithm value). Panel C shows the effect of the PAM on the dose–response curve to the agonist. It can be seen that potentiation occurs (the agonist dose–response curve shifts to the left) as reflected by the decrease in k_2. In this experiment, the rate of association (k_1) does not change.

reflect decreases in k_2, as k_1 is often diffusion rate-limited (see Fig. 5.11). Similarly, allosteric antagonism can result from either a decrease in k_1 or an increase in k_2; Fig. 5.12 shows the effect of increasing k_2 by a factor of five to produce a five-fold shift to the right of the agonist dose–response curve. The important concept in kinetic studies is the fact that a molecule

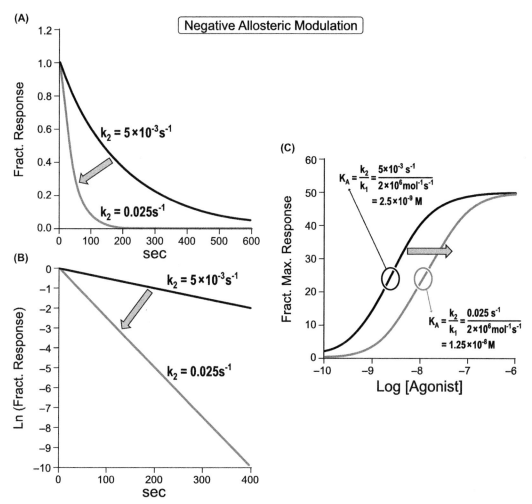

FIGURE 5.12 Alteration of kinetics of receptor dissociation by negative allosteric modulator. Panel A shows the offset of receptor response to an agonist in the presence of a high concentration of a competitive antagonist; this reversal of response reflects the rate of dissociation of the agonist from the receptor (k_2). The black line represents the system in the absence of the allosteric modulator; the gray line shows the increase in the offset rate (and subsequent increase in the rate of dissociation) in the presence of the negative allosteric modulator. It can be seen that the k_2 value increases by a factor of 5. Panel B shows the same plot on a log ordinate scale (fractional response expressed as the natural logarithm value). Panel C shows the effect of the allosteric modulator on the dose–response curve to the agonist. It can be seen that antagonism occurs (the agonist dose–response curve shifts to the right) as reflected by the increase in k_2. In this experiment, the rate of association (k_1) does not change.

must allow the agonist (probe of the receptor function) to bind in order to measure a change in rate of association or dissociation. Therefore, by definition, only an allosteric molecule can alter the kinetics of agonist binding; an orthosteric molecule binds to the same site as the agonist and therefore does not allow agonist binding.

QUANTIFYING ALLOSTERIC EFFECT

As with antagonism (see Chapter 4), allosteric effects can be quantified by comparing dose–response curves obtained in the presence of varying concentrations of allosteric modulators to behavior predicted by quantitative models. The model that will be used is given below showing receptors (R), a receptor probe agonist (A) and an allosteric modulator (B):

$$(5.1)$$

Allosteric modification of the effect is quantified by two co-operativity factors, namely α and β. The term α quantifies the effect of the modulator B on the affinity of the receptor to A (and similarly the reciprocal effect A has on the affinity of B). The term β quantifies the effect the modulator has on the efficacy of A. It can be seen from this model that an allosteric modulator cannot be characterized only by affinity (K_B^{-1}), but rather will also have a type of "efficacy" for the receptor and its interaction with A in the form of α and β. Accordingly, the following equation defines the response to an agonist (A) in the presence of an allosteric modulator (B) (see Derivations and Proofs, Appendix B8):[8]

Response =

$$\frac{(\tau_A[A](K_B + \alpha\beta[B]))^n\ E_m}{(\tau_A[A](K_B + \alpha\beta[B]))^n + ([A]K_B + K_AK_B + K_A[B] + \alpha[A][B])^n}$$

$$(5.2)$$

where E_m is the maximal response capability of the system, τ_A is the efficacy of the agonist, K_A

and K_B are the equilibrium dissociation constants of the agonist and modulator–receptor complexes respectively and n is a fitting factor for the curve. Just as for orthosteric antagonism, dose–response data is fit to equation 5.2 to yield values of K_B, α and β the characteristic descriptors of an allosteric modulator. For example, Fig. 5.13A shows the effects of an allosteric antagonist which decreases both affinity ($\alpha = 0.3$) and efficacy ($\beta = 0.2$) of the agonist. Figure 5.13B shows the effects of a positive allosteric modulator (PAM) that increases the affinity ($\alpha = 20$) and efficacy ($\beta = 2$) of the agonist.

Allosteric modulators stabilize conformational states of proteins and these may also have direct effects in their own right. Therefore, allosteric modulation can also be associated with direct agonism. Since a pure allosteric agonist binds to its own site on the protein and stabilizes an active state, this process can be independent of the process of natural agonism produced by the endogenous agonist. The allosteric agonist may not interfere with the binding of the endogenous agonist, therefore the resulting allosteric agonism will be additive to endogenous agonism; an example of this effect is shown in Fig. 5.14. However, since allosterism may produce a global change in the protein conformation, there is no *a priori* reason why an allosteric agonist could not produce direct agonism along with a modified endogenous agonist response. Therefore, just as with allosteric antagonists or PAMs, these changes could involve affinity (α) and/or efficacy (β). The model for description of agonist response in the presence of an allosteric modulator that may also produce direct agonism is (see Derivations and Proofs, Appendix B9):[8]

Response =

$$\frac{(\tau_A[A](K_B + \alpha\beta[B]) + \tau_B[B]K_A)^n\ E_m}{(\tau_A[A](K_B + \alpha\beta[B]) + \tau_B[B]K_A)^n + ([A]K_B + K_AK_B + K_A[B] + \alpha[A][B])^n}$$

$$(5.3)$$

where the designations of the parameters are the same as for equation 5.2 with the addition

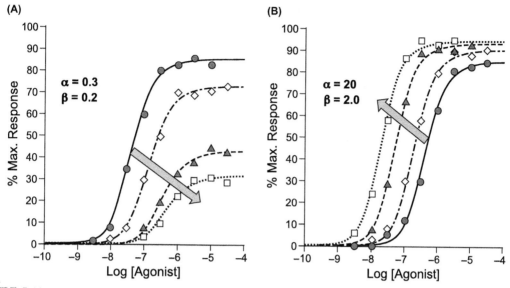

FIGURE 5.13 Fitting data to the model of allosteric function; Agonist $K_A = 300$ nM, $\tau = 3$, $E_m = 100$ (equation 5.2). Panel A: Antagonism fit to the model for a negative allosteric modulator of $K_B = 100$ nM, $\alpha = 0.3$, $\beta = 0.2$. Curves shown in the absence (filled circles) and presence of 300 nM (open diamonds), 2 μM (filled triangles) and 10 μM (open squares) negative modulator. Panel B: Data for a PAM of of $K_B = 100$ nM, $\alpha = 20$, $\beta = 2$. Curves shown in the absence (filled circles) and presence of 3 nM (open diamonds), 20 nM (filled triangles) and 100 nM (open squares) positive modulator.

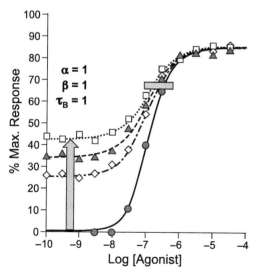

FIGURE 5.14 Fitting data to the model of allosteric function for modulator with direct agonist action for probe agonist $K_A = 300$ nM, $\tau = 3$, $E_m = 100$ (equation 5.3). Curves shown for the agonist alone and in the presence of an allosteric agonist of $K_B = 100$ nM, $\alpha = 1$, $\beta = 1$ and $\tau_B = 1$. Curves shown in the absence (filled circles) and presence of 100 nM (open diamonds), 200 nM (filled triangles) and 500 nM (open squares) allosteric agonist.

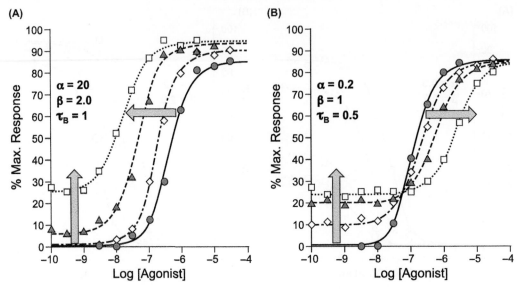

FIGURE 5.15. Fitting data to the model of allosteric function for modulator with direct agonist action. For control probe agonist $K_A = 300$ nM, $\tau = 3$, $E_m = 100$ (equation 5.3). Panel A: Data for a PAM-agonist of $K_B = 100$ nM, $\alpha = 20$, $\beta = 2$ and $\tau_B = 1$. Curves shown in the absence (filled circles) and presence of 3 nM (open diamonds), 20 nM (filled triangles) and 100 nM (open squares) PAM-agonist. Panel B: Antagonism fit to the model for a negative allosteric modulator with direct agonist activity of $K_B = 100$ nM, $\alpha = 0.3$, $\beta = 0.2$, $\tau_B = 0.5$. Curves shown in the absence (filled circles) and presence of 100 nM (open diamonds), 500 nM (filled triangles) and 3 µM (open squares) negative modulator-agonist.

that τ_B refers to the efficacy for direct agonism of the allosteric modulator. Figure 5.15A shows the effect of an allosteric agonist that also enhances the affinity ($\alpha = 20$) and efficacy ($\beta = 2$) of the endogenous agonist. It can be seen that in addition to a direct agonism, the responses to the endogenous agonist are enhanced. Figure 5.15B shows the effect of an allosteric agonist modulator that reduces the affinity of the endogenous agonist ($\alpha = 0.2$; with no effect on efficacy $\beta = 1$). Interestingly, this type of profile is very similar to that of a standard orthosteric partial agonist (see Fig. 4.19). To differentiate these profiles, the principles of saturation of effect and/or probe dependence would need to be applied.

The potency of an allosteric modulator is described by an affinity constant (pK_B) much like other antagonists. However, since allosteric systems describe the energy of interaction

between two molecules acting on the protein, the effective affinity of the modulator is modified by the α factor provided by the co-binding ligand. Under these circumstances, it can be seen that different α factors for different ligands can lead to varying affinity, i.e., the affinity of the modulator is contingent upon the nature of the co-binding ligand. Similarly, the functional effect of an allosteric modulator also depends upon the value of β, since this defines the effect of the modulator on the efficacy of the co-binding agonist. Therefore, to fully characterize the allosteric effect of a modulator, values for the pK_B, α, β and the identity of the co-binding must be designated. In practice, therapeutically targeted allosteric modulators usually deal with endogenous agonists; therefore a single set of pK_B, α and β values for the endogenous ligand may be sufficient for characterization. However, in the case of multiple endogenous ligands (such as for peptide receptors), complications may arise as the activity of the allosteric modulator may vary for different endogenous ligands. If probe dependence is *not* observed, it may be that the antagonist is still allosteric but that the wrong probes were utilized to detect the effect.

DESCRIPTIVE PHARMACOLOGY: V

A schematic diagram of the logic employed in the exploration of possible allosteric ligand effect is given in Fig. 5.16; it is governed by some key observations. The first observation describes the effect of the modulator on agonist response; if response is increased then an allosteric effect is assumed, since an orthosteric mechanism cannot accommodate this mechanism. Specifically, a molecule must co-bind with the agonist to cause its potentiation. Under these circumstances, the dose–response curves can be fit to the allosteric model,

specifically equation 5.2 if no direct modulator agonist activity is seen and equation 5.3 if it is. The analysis is less straightforward if antagonism is observed. Under these circumstances the decision points identifying allosterism are based on conditional yes/no values. Specifically, if a distinct effect is obtained then allosterism is identified; if it is not, then it will be ambiguous in that allosterism may or may not be operative. For antagonism, if probe dependence is observed (i.e., the modulator blocks the effects of one agonist more than another), then allosterism is identified and equations 5.2 and 5.3 can be applied. If no probe dependence is seen it may be that the allosteric effect (if the antagonist is allosteric) is identical for the probes chosen for study. The next decision point comes from the observation of surmountability, i.e., does the antagonist depress the maximal response? If not, then the antagonist is either an orthosteric simple competitive blocker or it is producing surmountable allosteric antagonism. Under these

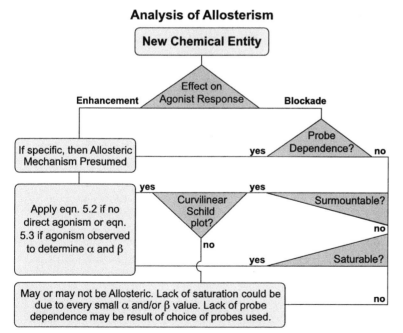

Analysis of Allosterism

FIGURE 5.16. Logic for determining whether the effect of a given ligand is allosteric — see text.

circumstances, the concentrations for blockade should be maximized to identify possible curvilinearity in the Schild plot (i.e., see Fig. 5.4B). If this is observed, allosterism is identified and equations 5.2 and 5.3 can be applied.

If depression of the maximal response is produced, then the concentrations of modulator can be increased to maximal values to try to identify saturation of effect (i.e., see Fig. 5.10B). If the antagonist brings the agonist maximal response to baseline, then either the molecule is a non-competitive orthosteric blocker or the values for β are small enough to completely negate agonism. If the depression of maximum reaches an asymptotic limit (Fig. 5.10B), then allosterism is identified and equations 5.2 or 5.3 can be applied.

of effect and/or probe dependence to identify allosteric mechanisms.
- Only allosteric modulators can affect the kinetics of association or dissociation of co-binding ligands.
- Once allosterism has been identified as a mechanism, then comparison of data to an allosteric model can be used to identify characteristic parameters of the effect.
- These characteristics are: α (the effect of the modulator on the affinity of the co-binding ligand) and β (the effect of the modulator on the efficacy of the co-binding ligand).
- The magnitude of the pK_B (equilibrium dissociation constant of the modulator receptor complex) will depend on the nature of the co-binding ligand.

SUMMARY

The following concepts are discussed in this chapter:

- Allosteric systems are permissive in that two ligands bind to a protein (each to their own separate binding site) and affect the reactivity of the protein to each.
- This co-binding mechanism imparts unique features to allosteric modulators due to three distinct properties.
- The first unique property of allosterism is *saturability of effect*, i.e., the allosteric modulation ends when the allosteric site is fully occupied.
- The second property is *probe dependence*, i.e., the allosteric effect of a given modulator can be different for different co-binding ligands.
- The third property is that allosteric modulation can induce *separate effects* on co-binding ligand *affinity* and *efficacy*.
- While allosteric antagonism can appear to be simple orthosteric blockade, experiments can be done to identify possible saturation

QUESTIONS

5.1 A given antagonist was found to produce potent surmountable blockade with a pA_2 value of 8.0. When investigators used 100 times the pA_2 concentration (10^{-6} M) in an attempt to completely block a process, they were surprised to find that the process was still not blocked and partially operative (only a four-fold shift of the curve appeared). What could be happening?

5.2 A discovery effort was aimed at potentiating insulin release through the GLP-1 receptor and accordingly, a screen was run to detect PAMs. To facilitate the mechanics of the screen, a stable analog of the natural agonist for the GLP-1 receptor, exendin, was used. Subsequent lead optimization of hits showed an alarming lack of correspondence of effect in a natural system of insulin release; why might this occur?

5.3 A given antagonism is found to produce a 50% depression of the maximal response to an agonist at a concentration of 10 nM. What experiments can be done to determine if this effect is steric blockade (orthosteric antagonism) or allosteric modulation?

5.4 The pK_B of an allosteric antagonist for a chemokine receptor was measured to be 8.2 for blocking the effects of the chemokine CCL5. However, as a blocker of CCL3 (a different chemokine) it was found to be 7.5. What could be causing this difference?

References

[1] D.E. Koshland, The active site of enzyme action, Adv. Enzymol. 22 (1960) 45–97.

[2] F. Monod, J. Wyman, J.P. Changeuz, On the nature of allosteric transitions, J. Biol. Chem. 12 (1965) 88–118.

[3] H.E. Umbarger, Evidence for a negative feedback mechanism in the biosynthesis of isoleucine, Science 123 (1956) 848.

[4] C. Watson, S. Jenkinson, W. Kazmierski, T.P. Kenakin, The CCR5 receptor-based mechanism of action of 873140, a potent allosteric non-competitive HIV entry-inhibitor, Mol. Pharmacol. 67 (2005) 1268–1282.

[5] V.M. Muniz-Medina, S. Jones, J.M. Maglich, C. Galardi, R.E. Hollingsworth, W.M. Kazmierski, et al., The relative activity of "function sparing" HIV-1 entry inhibitors on viral entry and CCR5 internalization: Is allosteric functional selectivity a valuable therapeutic property? Mol. Pharmacol. 75 (2009) 490–501.

[6] S. Suratman, K. Leach, P.M. Sexton, C.C. Felder, R.E. Loiacono, A. Christopoulos, Impact of species variability and "probe-dependence" on the detection and in vivo validation of allosteric modulation at the M4 muscarinic acetylcholine receptor, Br. J. Pharmacol. 162 (2011) 1659–1670.

[7] C. Koole, D. Wooten, J. Simms, C. Valant, R. Sridhar, O.L. Woodman, et al., Allosteric ligands of the glucagon-like peptide 1 receptor (GLP-1R) differentially modulate endogenous and exogenous peptide responses in a pathway-selective manner: Implications for drug screening, Mol. Pharmacol. 78 (2010) 456–465.

[8] K. Leach, P.M. Sexton, A. Christopoulos, Allosteric GPCR modulators: Taking advantage of permissive receptor pharmacology, Trends Pharmacol. Sci. 28 (2007) 382–389.

[9] J.N.C. Kew, G. Trube, J.A. Kemp, A novel mechanism of activity-dependent NMDA receptor antagonism describes the effect of ifenprodil in rat cultured cortical neurons, J. Physiol. 497(3) (1996) 761–772.

[10] M.R. Price, G.L. Baillie, A. Thomas, L.A. Stevenson, M. Easson, R. Goodwin, et al., Allosteric modulation of the cannabinoid CB1 receptor, Mol. Pharmacol. 68 (2005) 1484–1495.

6

Enzymes as Drug Targets

By the end of this chapter students will understand how enzymes can be therapeutic drug targets. In addition, the four basic mechanisms of reversible enzyme inhibition, the topic of irreversible enzyme inhibition and enzyme activation will be discussed. Finally, the special cases of drug action on intracellular enzymes will be considered.

INTRODUCTION

Enzymes are nature's ubiquitous catalysts mediating thousands of biochemical reactions in the cell to control energy metabolism, oversee macromolecular synthesis and anabolic processes, regulate cell signaling and control cell cycles. Enzymes also control the level of critical molecules in the cell. They do this through accelerating the rate of chemical reactions by lowering the reaction activation energy. Without such catalysts these reactions would progress too slowly to sustain life. For example, without the presence of adenosine deaminase, the removal of the amine from adenosine would take 120 years (as opposed to the rate constant of activation of the enzyme of 370 seconds — an enhancement of 2.1×10^{12}-fold). Hundreds of enzymes control complex biochemical networks (many with strict fidelity to substrate type), although there are notable exceptions to this rule (see Box 6.1). Owing to their obvious key physiological role, enzymes are prime targets for therapeutic drug intervention.

NEW TERMINOLOGY

- **Catalysis**: The process of an enzyme producing a product from a bound substrate.

BOX 6.1

CYTOCHROME 3A4: NATURE'S PROMISCUOUS PROTECTOR

Most enzymes are conservative with respect to the substrate with which they interact so as to preserve signaling and biochemical fidelity in cell pathways. The cytochrome P450 enzymes, however, are designed to be promiscuous since their job is to protect the body from all foreign chemicals. In drug development, drugs are tested as possible inhibitors of cytochrome P450 enzymes as this could cause possible problematic drug–drug interactions. However, the promiscuity and different substrate handling of the most important cytochrome P450 enzyme, namely CYP3A4, can pose practical problems for prediction of such effects. For example, while quinidine makes no distinction between two substrates for CYP3A4 (BzRes = benzoyloxyresorufin and BQ = 7-benzyloxyquinoline), the drug astemizole does. Thus, the data with BQ shows astemizole to be a potent inhibitor of CYP3A4 (predicting drug–drug interactions) while the data with BzRes shows it to be relatively inactive (data from [5]).

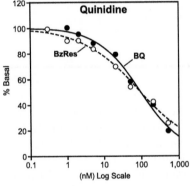
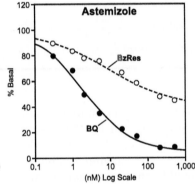

- **Competitive inhibition**: The inhibitor and substrate compete for the substrate binding site.
- **Covalent bond**: Chemical bond formed between the inhibitor and enzyme through alkylation.
- **Irreversible inhibition**: The inhibitor has a neglible rate of dissociation from the enzyme once it binds.
- **K_m**: Michaelis–Menten constant referring to the sensitivity of an enzyme to a given substrate; it encompasses substrate binding and catalysis.

- **Mechanism-based inhibition**: The enzyme creates an active species through catalysis which then goes on to alkylate the enzyme and inactivate it.
- **Mixed inhibition**: The inhibitor has different affinities for the enzyme and enzyme–substrate complex.
- **Non-competitive inhibition**: The inhibitor has equal affinity for the enzyme and the enzyme–substrate complex.
- **Substrate inhibition**: High concentrations of the substrate bind to different parts of the active site and enzyme activity is blocked.

- **Suicide inhibitor**: The inhibitor binds to the enzyme active site and irreversibly inactivates the enzyme when it does so.
- **Tight-binding inhibitor**: The inhibitor has a neglible rate of dissociation from the enzyme once it binds, although the bond between the inhibitor and enzyme may not be covalent.
- **Uncompetitive inhibition**: The inhibitor binds only to the enzyme–substrate complex.

- V_{max}: The maximal rate of enzyme hydrolysis (characteristic for an enzyme–substrate pair).

ENZYME KINETICS

The model used to describe enzyme kinetics is shown in Fig. 6.1A. Thus, a substrate binds to an enzyme (with a standard rate of association k_1 and dissociation k_2) and then a process

(A)

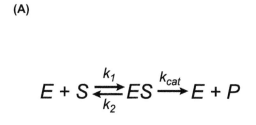

(B)

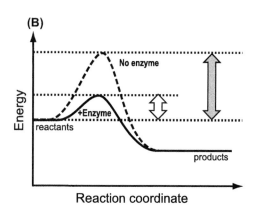

(C)

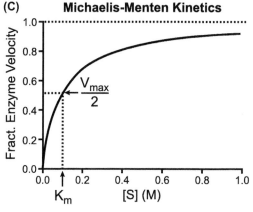

(D)

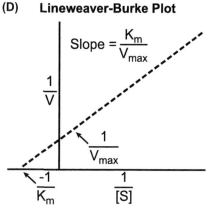

FIGURE 6.1   Enzyme catalysis. (A) Scheme showing substrate [S] binding to enzyme [E] to form a complex [ES] which then, through k_{cat}, converts substrate to product [P] and initiates regeneration of enzyme E. (B) This can be seen as the enzyme functioning as a catalyst to lower the energy barrier for production of the product. (C) Graphical representation of the Michaelis–Menten equation for enzyme function (equation 6.1). (D) Linear transformation of the Michaelis–Menten equation as published by Lineweaver and Burk (equation 6.3).

of catalysis occurs (with a new rate constant k_{cat}) which results in a product (formed from the substrate) and regeneration of the enzyme. The enzyme thus acts as a catalyst to reduce the energy barrier that separates the substrate from the product (Fig. 6.1B). Enzymes can modify a single molecule or catalyze a reaction between two molecules; this can form a single product or there can be an exchange of atoms to produce two or more different products. The formal kinetic model used to describe enzyme reactions is the Michaelis—Menten model according to the equation (see Derivations and Proofs, Appendix B10):

$$\text{Velocity} = \frac{[S]V_{max}}{[S] + K_m} \quad (6.1)$$

where [S] is the substrate concentration. V_{max} is the maximal rate of enzyme reaction and this, along with the magnitude of the amount of enzyme in the cell (and where it is located) describes the capacity of the enzyme system for catalysis. The K_m is a constant describing the sensitivity of the enzyme reaction to substrate. In molecular terms, the K_m is further defined (see Fig. 6.1A) as:

$$K_m = \frac{k_2 + k_{cat}}{k_1} \quad (6.2)$$

The affinity of the substrate for the enzyme is described (as for binding in the Langmuir adsorption isotherm; see equation 2.1) as $K_d = k_2/k_1$, but since this isn't a static binding process (the reaction continues to formation of product), k_{cat} must be included to describe the influence of catalysis on the binding process; k_{cat} is the collective rate constant for the forward progress of the chemical steps in catalysis. Therefore, K_d does not equal K_m unless $k_{cat} \ll k_2$.

Figure 6.1C shows a graphical representation of equation 6.1; there are notable features in this relationship. For low substrate concentrations, enzyme velocity $\rightarrow (k_{cat}/K_m)[E][S]$ where [E] is the enzyme concentration. Thus the velocity of the reaction depends upon both the substrate concentration and the amount of enzyme present. Under these circumstances the reaction resembles a bi-molecular reaction with a pseudo second-order rate constant of k_{cat}/K_m. Efficient enzymes have values of k_{cat}/K_m approaching 10^8 to $10^{10}\,M^{-1}\,s^{-1}$ (this becomes diffusion-limited). With high substrate concentrations ([S]$\gg$$K_m$) the enzyme velocity is $V_{max} = k_{cat}[E]$. Under these circumstances the rate of reaction depends only on the amount of enzyme present (unimolecular reaction with pseudo first-order rate constant k_{cat}).

The graphical relationship between substrate concentration and enzyme velocity according to the Michaelis—Menten equation (equation 6.1) is shown in Fig. 6.1C. Here it can be seen that the maximal velocity is V_{max} and the half-maximal velocity is the K_m (as a substrate concentration). Historically, a linear double reciprocal metameter of equation 6.1 has been used to analyze enzyme reactions according to the equation:

$$\frac{1}{V} = \frac{K_m}{[S]V_{max}} + \frac{1}{V_{max}} \quad (6.3)$$

Termed the Lineweaver—Burk equation, this yields a straight line with abscissal intercept of $-1/K_m$, an ordinate intercept of $1/V_{max}$ and a slope of K_m/V_{max} (see Fig. 6.1D). Before the widespread availability of computers able to fit data directly to non-linear functions, linear transformations such as the Lineweaver—Burk plot were used to estimate parameters; these could be calculated through linear regressional analysis. However, the availability of techniques to fit data directly to the Michaelis—Menten equation has supplanted the use of linear transformations as the latter, being double reciprocal plots, can lead to seriously skewed estimates of parameters and are highly unreliable for the estimation of enzyme constants. It will be seen in future sections, however, that the Lineweaver—Burk plot can still be useful as an identifier of type of enzyme inhibition.

ENZYMES AS DRUG TARGETS

Enzyme inhibitors have been used as therapeutic drugs throughout pharmacological history (see Box 6.2). There are numerous scenarios where drug intervention into an enzyme reaction can yield therapeutically favorable outcomes. These are:

1. **Enzyme inhibition to alter levels of normal physiological cellular molecules**. For example, the enzyme phosphodiesterase degrades the physiologically active second messenger cyclic AMP in cardiac cells; this controls cardiac contractility and sinus rhythm. In failing hearts (congestive heart failure), a useful augmentation of contractility can be obtained by blockade of enzymatic degradation of cyclic AMP; phosphodiesterase inhibitors such as milrinone are useful in congestive heart failure. Augmentation of cardiac contractility can also be gained from blockade of ATPase enzymes in heart muscle (e.g., using digitalis) and erectile dysfunction can be treated by blockade of cyclic GMP degradation by phosphodiesterase V inhibition (sildenafil).

2. **Blockade of enzyme activity that becomes pathophysiological**. The renin–angiotensin system is intimately involved in blood pressure and fluid balance, and in conditions

---

BOX 6.2

FROM BITTER BARK TO A UNIVERSAL REMEDY

From the time of Hippocrates, (circa 460 BC to 377 BC) extracts from the bitter bark and leaves of the willow tree were known to alleviate pain and fever. In 1828, a Professor of Pharmacy at the University of Munich isolated a tiny amount of yellow needle-like crystalline bitter-tasting crystals from willow bark he called salicin. In 1897, chemists at Bayer AG led by Arthur Eichengrún and Felix Hoffmann produced acetylsalicylic acid from salicin. Hoffmann gave the new compound to his father who was suffering from arthritis and noticed an improvement. The compound was patented in 1900, named "Aspirin" (the "A" from acetyl and spir from *Spiraea ulmaria*, the plant from which it was derived).

Long thought to act through the central nervous system, John Vane and Priscilla Piper tested aspirin at the Royal College of Surgeons in London and noted that it blocked the production of what later were found to be prostaglandins. Subsequent research showed that aspirin is an irreversible inhibitor of the enzyme cyclooxygenase through acetylation of a serine residue at the active site. This gives the molecule its analgesic, anti-inflammatory and antipyretic activity.

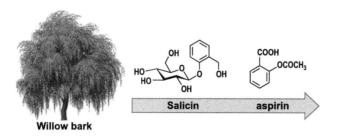

Willow bark

Salicin → aspirin

of hypertension, blockade of the angiotensin-converting enzyme (ACE) by drugs such as lisinopril lowers blood pressure. Similarly, aspirin blocks the enzyme cyclooxygenase to prevent formation of inflammatory prostaglandins and thromboxane (see Box 6.2). Inhibitors of xanthine oxidase prevent this enzyme from producing excess amounts of uric acid in gout.

3. **Blockade of an enzyme that exclusively takes part in a pathophysiological process**. After HIV infection and in the progression process to AIDS, HIV-1 utilizes the enzyme HIV reverse transcriptase to catalyze the production of viral DNA from the viral RNA template to facilitate further infection; drugs such as AZT (azidothymidine) effectively block this process. Penicillin is a suicide substrate that selectively blocks the enzyme that controls bacterial wall integrity to selectively destroy bacteria with no harm to the host (see Box 6.3). Similarly sulfa drugs such as sulfanilamide block dihydropteroate synthetase to prevent bacteria from synthesizing required folic acid; this is lethal to bacteria but not humans, providing a useful selective bacteriostatic action.

4. **Blockade of hyperactivity from enzymes**. Enzyme inhibitors can be selectively lethal to cells with varying levels of metabolic activity. For example, blockade of nucleotide synthesis by drugs such as methotrexate can be selectively lethal to rapidly growing cells carrying out DNA replication in tumors. In human breast cell tumors, the over-expression of HER2 can be countered by blockers of tyrosine kinase ErbB2 such as herceptin.

There are many drugs that have inhibition of enzymes as their mechanism of action (see Table 6.1).

BOX 6.3

PENICILLIN: LIFE SAVING SUICIDE SUBSTRATE

Penicillins are molecules produced by molds in the Penicillium family. Their antibiotic activity was discovered in 1928 by Alexander Fleming, but penicillins were not widely used therapeutically until the 1940s. Penicillins act as suicide substrates of glycopeptide transpeptidase in bacteria. Thus, penicillin enters the active site as a substrate, but in the normal process of catalysis forms a covalent bond to permanently inactive the enzyme. This enzyme is essential for bacterial wall cross-linking, thus inactivation by penicillin disrupts bacterial integrity and causes death. There is no corresponding process in humans, therefore the biochemical reaction is unique to bacteria; this makes penicillin a valuable antibiotic. Some bacteria have developed penicillin resistance through expression of an enzyme β-lactamase. This enzyme opens the four-membered ring of penicillins.

TABLE 6.1 Some Drugs Targeted for Enzymes

Compound	Target Enzyme	Disease (Indication)
Acetazolamine	Carbonic anhydrase	Glaucoma
Acyclovir	Viral DNA polymerase	Herpes
Agenerase	Viral protease	AIDS
Amprenavir	HIV protease	AIDS
Allopurinol	Xanthine oxidase	Gout
Argatroban	Thrombin	Cardiovascular disease
Aspirin	Cyclooxygenase	Inflammation/pain/fever
Amoxicillin	Penicillin binding proteins	Bacterial infection
Carbidopa	Dopa decarboxylase	Parkinson's disease
Celebrex	Cyclooxygenase-2	Inflammation/pain/fever
Clavulanate	β-lactamase	Bacterial resistance
Combivir	Viral reverse transcriptase	AIDS
Digoxin	Na^+/K^+ ATPase	Congestive heart failure
Dutasteride	5-α-reductase	Benign prostate hyperplasia
Efavirenz	HIV reverse transcriptase	AIDS
Epristeride	Steroid 5-α-reductase	Benign prostate hyperplasia
Etopiside	Topoisomerase II	Cancer
Flurouracil	Thymidylate synthase	Cancer
Leflunomide	Dihydroorotate dehydrogenase	Inflammation
Levitra	Phosphodiesterase V	Erectile dysfunction
Lisinopril	Angiotensin converting enzyme	Hypertension
Lovastin	HMG-CoA reductase	Cardiovascular disease
Methotrexate	Dihydrofolate reductase	Cancer, immunosupression
Nitecapone	Catechol-o-methyl transferase	Parkinson's disease
Norflaxin	DNA gyrase	Urinary tract infection
Ompremazole	H^+/K^+ ATPase	Peptic ulcer
PALA	Aspartate transcarbamoylase	Cancer
Raltegravir	Viral integrase	AIDS
Relenza	Viral neurominidase	Influenza
Sorbinol	Aldose reductase	Diabetic retinopathy

(Continued)

TABLE 6.1 (Continued)

Compound	Target Enzyme	Disease (Indication)
Tacrine	Acetylcholinesterase	Alzheimer's disease
Trazodone	Adenosine deaminase	Depression
Trimethoprim	Bacterial dihydrofolate reductase	Bacterial infection
Tykerb	ErbB-2/EGFR	Breast cancer

REVERSIBLE ENZYME INHIBITION

The primary assumption for reversible enzyme inhibition is that the inhibitor binds to the enzyme through mass action, but that the binding can be reversed upon washing the enzyme with inhibitor free media, i.e., the inhibition is reversible. In general, there are two basic enzyme species to which an inhibitor could bind to produce enzyme inhibition; the enzyme not bound by substrate (E in Fig. 6.2) and the substrate bound species (ES in Fig. 6.2). Combinations of affinities for these two species lead to the four general behaviors of enzyme inhibitors; competitive, non-competitive, uncompetitive and mixed (see Fig. 6.2). In order of increasing affinity of the inhibitor for the ES species:

1. **Competitive inhibition**: This is where the inhibitor competes for the substrate at the substrate binding site. An example of a competitive inhibitor is ritonavir, an HIV protease inhibitor. This antagonist contains three peptide bonds and resembles the protein substrate for HIV protease. Competitive inhibitors have virtually no affinity for the ES species since the substrate already occupies their binding site when bound ($K_1 <<< K_2$ in Fig. 6.2). Therefore, the inhibitor increases K_m but does not change V_{max}; the equation for enzyme velocity in the presence of a competitive inhibitor is shown in Fig. 6.2. The effect of a competitive antagonist on an enzyme velocity curve is shown in Fig. 6.3A and in the Lineweaver–Burk format in Fig. 6.3B. An example of competitive inhibition in a therapeutic setting is given in Box 6.4.

2. **Mixed inhibition**: This is where the inhibitor has affinity for both the E and ES form but these affinities are not identical ($K_1 \neq K_2$; Fig. 6.2). In this type of inhibition, the inhibitor can bind to the ES form of the enzyme but its affinity for the enzyme is altered when the substrate is bound. Under most circumstances, this type of inhibition is allosteric (see Chapter 5) in that the inhibitor binds to a site different from that of the substrate. Mixed inhibitors interfere with substrate binding (thus increasing K_m) and also hamper catalysis (decreasing V_{max}). The effect of a mixed antagonist on enzyme velocity is shown in Fig. 6.4A and in the Lineweaver–Burk format in Fig. 6.4B.

3. **Non-competitive inhibition**: In this form of enzyme inhibition, the inhibitor has the same affinity for E and ES, does not affect the binding of the substrate ($K_1 = K_2$ in Fig. 6.2), but does reduce catalysis. Therefore, there is no effect on the K_m but the V_{max} for the reaction is decreased; the equation for non-competitive antagonism is shown in Fig. 6.2. The effect of a non-competitive antagonist on enzyme velocity is shown in Fig. 6.5A and in the Lineweaver–Burk format in Fig. 6.5B. An example of a non-competitive inhibitor for an enzyme is shown by the effects of Efavirenz on HIV Reverse Transcriptase.

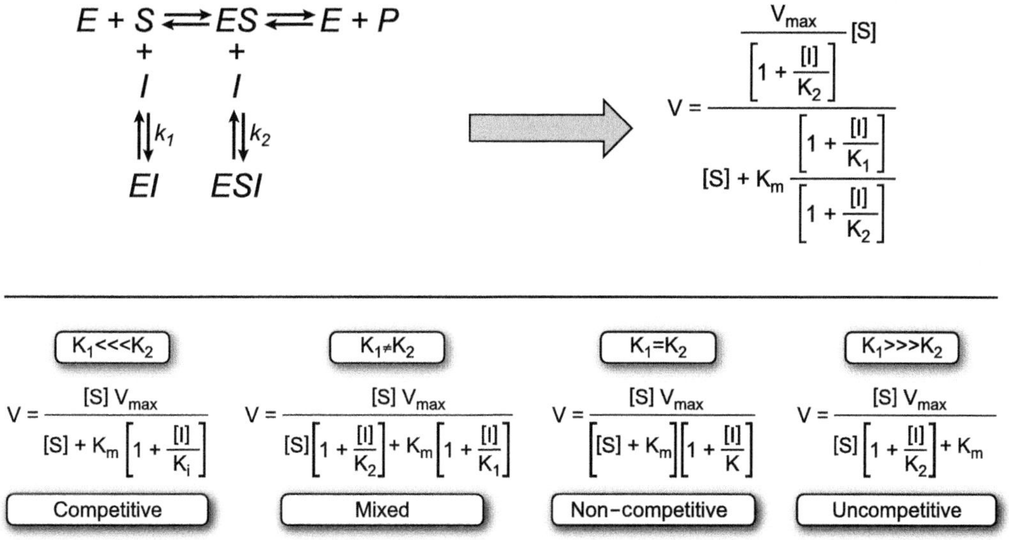

$$E + S \rightleftharpoons ES \rightleftharpoons E + P$$

$$V = \dfrac{\dfrac{V_{max}}{\left[1 + \dfrac{[I]}{K_2}\right]}[S]}{[S] + K_m \dfrac{\left[1 + \dfrac{[I]}{K_1}\right]}{\left[1 + \dfrac{[I]}{K_2}\right]}}$$

$E + S \rightleftharpoons ES$ with $+ I$ below each (with k_1 forming EI and k_2 forming ESI)

$K_1 <<< K_2$	$K_1 \neq K_2$	$K_1 = K_2$	$K_1 >>> K_2$
$V = \dfrac{[S]\,V_{max}}{[S] + K_m\left[1 + \dfrac{[I]}{K_i}\right]}$	$V = \dfrac{[S]\,V_{max}}{[S]\left[1 + \dfrac{[I]}{K_2}\right] + K_m\left[1 + \dfrac{[I]}{K_1}\right]}$	$V = \dfrac{[S]\,V_{max}}{\left[[S] + K_m\right]\left[1 + \dfrac{[I]}{K}\right]}$	$V = \dfrac{[S]\,V_{max}}{[S]\left[1 + \dfrac{[I]}{K_2}\right] + K_m}$
Competitive	Mixed	Non-competitive	Uncompetitive

FIGURE 6.2 Schematic of the binding of inhibitors to various forms of the enzyme; either free enzyme [E] or the enzyme—substrate complex [ES]. The general equation for the inhibitor binding to the two forms of the enzyme is shown in the box to the right, with K_1 and K_2 describing interactions of inhibitor with E and ES respectively. Various relationships between K_1 and K_2 lead to four basic mechanisms of enzyme inhibition: competitive; mixed; non-competitive and uncompetitive (see text).

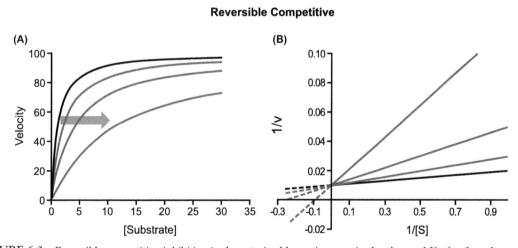

Reversible Competitive

FIGURE 6.3 Reversible competitive inhibition is characterized by an increase in the observed K_m for the substrate and no diminution of V_{max}. The Lineweaver—Burk plots are of increasing slope (indicating increasing values of K_m) with higher levels of inhibitor, and intersect at the ordinate axis. The enzyme inhibitor has negligible affinity for ES since the substrate impedes binding to the ES species.

BOX 6.4

A LIFE-SAVING COMPETITION

Methanol is extremely toxic due to central nervous system depression and through production of formate via the enzyme alcohol dehydrogenase. Formate is made from formaldehyde and is toxic to mitochondrial cytochrome c oxidase. This leads to symptoms of hypoxia, metabolic acidosis and other metabolic disturbances. Treatment is through competitive inhibition of the enzymatic reaction using an excess of ethanol or fomepizole. These molecules compete for methanol at the active site of alcohol dehydrogenase and formaldehyde production is halted.

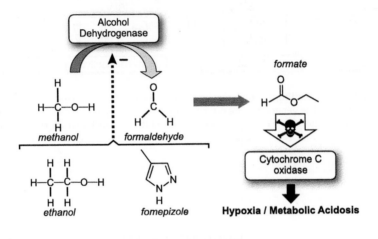

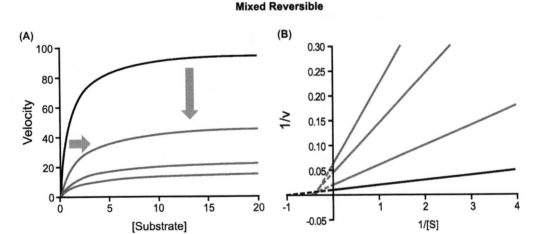

FIGURE 6.4   Mixed inhibition is characterized by increasing K_m values and decreasing apparent V_{max}. The enzyme inhibitor has an unequal affinity for E and ES.

Non–competitive Reversible

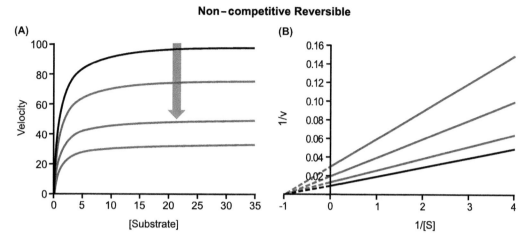

FIGURE 6.5 Non-competitive inhibition is characterized by no change in the K_m value and a decrease in V_{max}. The enzyme inhibitor has an equal affinity for both E and ES.

4. **Uncompetitive inhibition**: This is where the inhibitor binds only to the ES enzyme–substrate complex and not to the enzyme with no substrate bound ($K_1 >>> K_2$; Fig. 6.2). Under these circumstances, V_{max} is decreased but the apparent K_m will decrease as well due to the selective binding of the inhibitor to the ES species. In essence the binding of the substrate creates the binding site for the inhibitor; therefore, the binding of the inhibitor is promoted by the presence of the substrate. The effect of an uncompetitive antagonist on enzyme velocity is shown in Fig. 6.6A and in the Lineweaver–Burk format in Fig. 6.6B. A special case of uncompetitive inhibition is substrate inhibition whereby the substrate itself blocks enzyme activity at high concentrations. This is caused by more than one substrate molecule binding to the active site of the enzyme meant for just one substrate molecule, e.g., different parts of the substrate molecule bind to different parts of the enzyme active site. Thus, the counterpart for the inhibitor species in Fig. 6.2 is ESS. An example of this type of effect is demonstrated by sucrose at the enzyme invertase. The equation for substrate

inhibition is a variant of the equation for uncompetitive inhibition:

$$V = \frac{[S]V_{max}}{[S]\left[1 + \frac{[S]}{K_S}\right] + K_m} \tag{6.4}$$

where K_S is the affinity of the substrate for the enzyme with another substrate molecule already bound.

The mechanism of enzyme inhibition can be important since it may define the relationship between the inhibitor concentrations needed to produce blockade and the level of substrate present in the enzyme compartment. For example, high substrate levels make a competitive inhibitor less potent but an uncompetitive inhibitor more potent. While a detailed analysis of the effects of inhibitors on enzyme activation curves (or an analysis of Lineweaver–Burk curves) can yield information on the mechanism of inhibition, another relatively simple approach is to quantify the relationship between the IC_{50} (molar concentration producing 50% inhibition of enzyme activity) and the K_i. Figure 6.7 shows the relationship between the IC_{50} of the four types of inhibitor and the level of substrate. The equations relating the IC_{50} and K_i are given in Table 6.2.

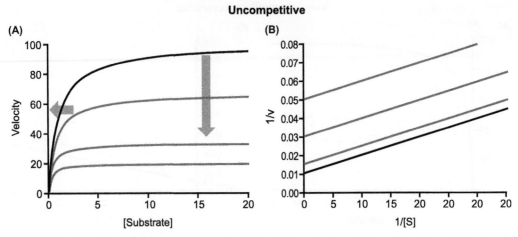

FIGURE 6.6 Uncompetitive inhibition is characterized by a decrease in the apparent K_m value and a decreased V_{max}. The Lineweaver–Burk plots are parallel and do not intersect. The enzyme inhibitor has neglible affinity for E but a high affinity for the enzyme–substrate complex (ES).

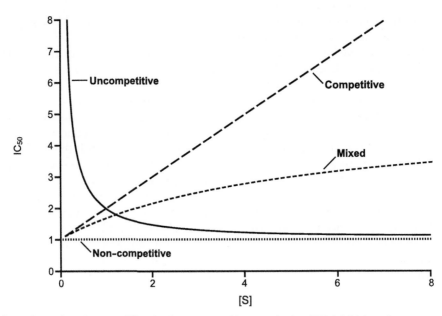

FIGURE 6.7 Relationships between IC_{50}s (molar concentrations producing 50% inhibition of an enzyme reaction run at a defined substrate concentration) and the substrate concentration. The potency of non-competitive inhibitors is independent of substrate concentration, whereas a linear relationship defines competitive inhibition. A non-linear relationship exists for mixed inhibitors (the extent of the non-linearity depends on differences between K_1 and K_2). Uncompetitive inhibitors become more potent with increasing substrate concentration.

TABLE 6.2 Relationship Between IC_{50} and K_i for Various Types of Enzyme Inhibition

Description	IC_{50}/K_i Relationship
Competitive inhibition	$K_i = \dfrac{IC_{50}}{\left[1 + \frac{[S]}{K_m}\right]}$
Mixed inhibition	$K_i = \dfrac{IC_{50}}{\left[\frac{K_m}{K_1} + \frac{[S]}{K_2}\right]}$
Non-competitive inhibtion	$K_i = IC_{50}$
Uncompetitive inhibition	$K_i = \dfrac{IC_{50}}{\left[1 + \frac{K_m}{[S]}\right]}$

IRREVERSIBLE ENZYME INHIBITION

Useful therapeutic effects can also be obtained from irreversible inhibition of enzyme function. These molecules do not dissociate (or dissociate extremely slowly) from the enzyme. An inhibitor can produce essentially irreversible inhibition through the induction of a conformational change in the enzyme to form a highly stabilized complex. Such "tight binding" inhibitors can be useful therapeutic agents since they have K_i values typically less than 5 nM; only very low concentrations of these are required for enzyme inhibition, thereby yielding considerable selectivity. An example of such a tight binding inhibitor is shown in Fig. 6.8; Immucillin H blocks purine nucleoside phosphorylase irreversibly with extremely high potency.

Given sufficient time, an irreversible inhibitor will eventually inactivate all of the enzyme present until the velocity of the enzyme reaction is zero. Since irreversible molecules do not come to equilibrium with their targets, the standard techniques to measure the potency of such molecules cannot be used; other methods are required. One example of this type of procedure is shown in Fig. 6.8. Specifically, this figure shows one approach whereby a concentration of irreversible inactivator is added to an enzyme preparation and the amount of product measured with time; it can be seen that eventually there is no further product formed as the enzyme becomes completely inactivated. The initial slope of this curve can yield a measure of the initial enzyme velocity v_i which, for a one-step inactivation process, can be used to estimate a k_{obs} according to the equation:

$$[Product]_{time} = \frac{v_i}{k_{obs}}(1 - e^{-k_{obs}t}) \qquad (6.5)$$

A subsequent plot of various k_{obs} values with different concentrations of irreversible inhibitor yields a measure of $k_{obs}/[I]$ (from the slope of a regression of K_{obs} on [A]) which can be used to quantify irreversible inhibitor activity.

A common mechanism for irreversible enzyme blockade is alkylation where a covalent bond is formed with the protein (or one of its bound co-factors). An example of this type of effect is shown by diisopropylflurophosphonate alkylation of acetylcholinesterase. If an inhibitor forms a covalent bond it usually means that a reactive species is involved and this can lead to problems with specificity, as a reactive species may alkylate a range of proteins in addition to the enzyme. One mechanism whereby an alkylating agent can be more specific is in the case of suicide substrates. These bind specifically to the active site and while bound are in a favorable orientation to alkylate; and example of such an agent is penicillin (see Box 6.3). The enzyme could also act on an initially non-reactive molecule to produce a reactive species which then goes on to alkylate the enzyme; this is referred to as mechanism-based inhibition. This is often seen with hepatic cytochrome P450 enzymes designed to attack foreign molecules in the liver (see Chapter 7). Figure 6.9 shows mechanism-based inhibition of CYP2C9 by erythromycin characterized by an inordinately long onset to steady-state effect. Usually in these cases, the only way to regenerate the enzyme activity is to synthesize new enzyme.

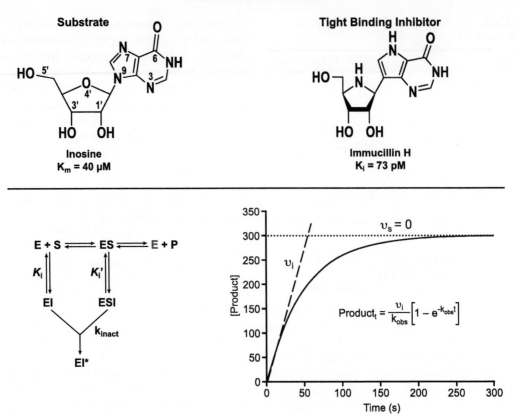

FIGURE 6.8 Irreversible enzyme inhibition. Top panel: Example of a tight binding inhibitor. The substrate for purine nucleoside phosphorylase is inosine; Immucillin H is an extremely potent and irreversible inhibitor although no covalent bond is formed. Bottom panels: The scheme for irreversible enzyme inhibition is shown on the left while a method for estimating the activity of an irreversible inhibitor is shown on the right. In this procedure, the kinetics of production of product, from a given concentration of substrate, is observed in the presence of an irreversible inhibitor. A tangent depicts v_i which is then used to estimate k_{obs}, a measure of inhibition. Values of k_{obs} for different substrate concentrations can be used to obtain a general parameter characterizing the activity of the irreversible inhibitor (see text).

Enzyme Activation

Enzyme activation can be accelerated through biochemical modification of the enzyme (i.e., phosphorylation) or through low molecular weight positive modulators. Just as with agonists of receptors, it is theoretically possible to bind molecules to enzymes to increase catalysis (enzyme activators). These molecules must bind to a site other than the substrate binding site, otherwise substrate binding cannot occur. There are conditions where enzyme activators could be of benefit therapeutically. For instance, activators of glucokinase that increase the sensitivity of the enzyme to glucose could cause an increased insulin secretion and liver glycogen synthesis, and decreased liver glucose output in diabetes (see Fig. 6.10).[1] Identification of enzyme activators requires correct configuration of the assay (e.g., low substrate concentration) since most enzyme assays are designed to detect inhibitors.

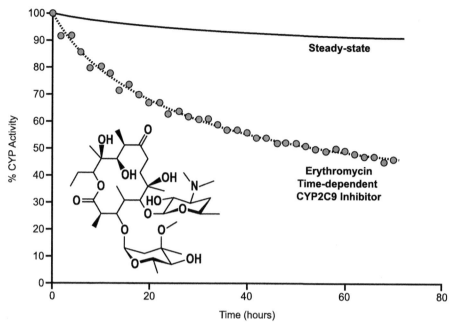

FIGURE 6.9 Time-dependent (mechanism-based) enzyme inhibition of cytochrome 2C9 by erythromycin. While a reversible inhibitor comes to equilibrium or steady-state within a few hours, time-dependent inhibition continues over an extremely long period as the inhibitor slowly (and irreversibly) binds to the enzyme and inactivates it (data from [3]).

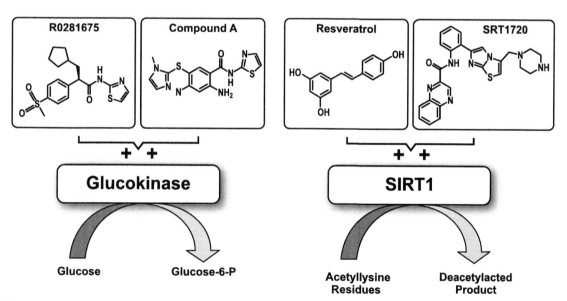

FIGURE 6.10 Enzyme activators. The production of glucose-6-phosphate from glucose is accelerated by RO281675 (data from [4]) and compound A, while Sirt1 production of deacylated products from acetyllysine residues is promoted by Resveratrol and SRT1720 (data from [1]).

INTRACELLULAR EFFECTS OF ENZYME-ACTIVE DRUGS

While enzymes can readily be assayed in biochemical assays where the concentration of substrate and inhibitor is known, most therapeutic enzyme inhibitors must access the enzyme in the cell. There are two elements important to assessing enzyme effects in cells; the level of endogenous basal enzyme activity and the concentrations of inhibitor that can access the enzyme in the cell. First to be considered is the level of basal enzyme activity as this controls the observed consequence of enzyme inhibition in the therapeutic setting.

The inhibition of a pathologically-linked enzyme may not lead to excitation of a target protein, but may nevertheless lead to a therapeutic effect. Endogenous basal activity can be very important to the inhibition of enzymes for therapeutic effect, since the magnitude of the observed effect depends directly on the endogenous tone of the system mediated by the enzyme. An example is the positive inotropic effects of phosphodiesterase (PDE) inhibitors in the treatment of congestive heart failure. In cardiac muscle, contractility is mediated by intracellular levels of cyclic AMP and these levels are tightly controlled by PDE-mediated hydrolysis. Therefore, blockade of PDE leads to a relaxation of this control and an excess of cyclic AMP; this leads to a positive stimulation of cardiac muscle. In the absence of basal cyclic AMP production in cardiac muscle, a PDE inhbitor will have no stimulant effect on the heart. It is useful to discuss the interplay between the basal activity of such systems and the observed response *in vivo*.

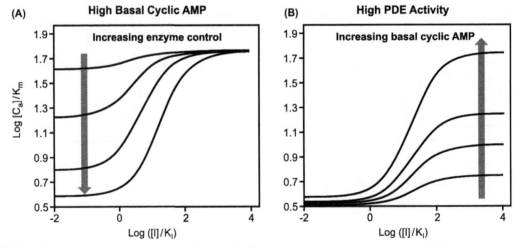

FIGURE 6.11 Effects of *in vivo* enzyme inhibition. (A) Dose–response curve of an enzyme inhibitor in systems where the ambient basal level of substrate is high. The range of curves result from various systems where the enzyme V_{max} is low (ordinate value is highest basal level of second messenger, $[C_a]/K_m = 1.64$) to high (ordinate value is basal = 0.58). Note how the effects of the enzyme inhibitor are more pronounced in the system where the enzyme V_{max} is high, indicating that it is an important control of cellular second messenger levels. (B) Effects of an enzyme inhibitor for an enzyme of high activity in cells of varying levels of basal second messenger. Note how the effects of enzyme inhibitor are more pronounced in systems with high levels of second messenger.

One solution for the equation linking second messenger levels in cells and enzyme activity is:[2]

$$\frac{[C_a]}{[K_m]} = \frac{1}{2}\left(\frac{[C_b]}{[K_m]} - \frac{V_{max}}{K_t \bullet K_m} - \frac{[I]}{K_I}\right)$$
$$+ \frac{1}{2}\sqrt{\left(1 + \frac{[I]}{K_I} + \frac{V_{max}}{K_t \bullet K_m} - \frac{[C_b]}{K_m}\right)^2 + \frac{[C_b]}{K_m}\left(1 + \frac{[I]}{K_I}\right)}$$

(6.6)

where $[C_b]$ and $[C_a]$ refer to the concentrations of cyclic AMP at the site of production (adenylate cyclase) and site of utilization (protein kinase) respectively, and k_t is an intracellular transfer rate constant between the two compartments. K_I is the equilibrium dissociation constant of the PDE-inhibitor enzyme complex,

K_m is the concentration of cyclic AMP where hydrolysis is half-maximal and V_{max} is the maximal rate of cyclic AMP hydrolysis.

This equation generally describes the effect of an enzyme inhibitor on free intracellular second messenger levels. It can be seen that a difference in second messenger levels (leading to a physiological effect) can be achieved if there is a high production of second messenger that is reduced by a high level of enzyme activity. Figure 6.11A shows the effect of basal enzyme activity on the observed dose–response curve to an enzyme inhibitor; it can be seen that if the enzyme activity is low (low level of $V_{max}/k_t \bullet K_m$) then the high basal second messenger levels are not further increased by the enzyme inhibitor. In

---

BOX 6.5

ENZYME BLOCKADE BECOMES RELEVANT WHEN THE ENZYME BEGINS TO WORK

Elevated levels of the second messenger cyclic AMP increase myocardial contractility, but in normal physiology the enzyme phosphodiesterase keeps cellular cylic AMP levels low. The phosphodiesterase inhibitor fenoximone blocks phosphophodiesterase to cause elevated levels of cyclic AMP, resulting in positive myocardial contractility. This can be beneficial for a failing heart in congestive heat failure (CHF) and fenoximone improves contractility in models of CHF *in vivo*. However, fenoximone has no effect *in vitro* until cyclic AMP is artificially elevated (through addition of sub-threshold levels of catecholamines). This models the *in vivo* situation where natural sympathetic nervous system tone causes elevated cyclic AMP in heart muscle (data from [2,6]).

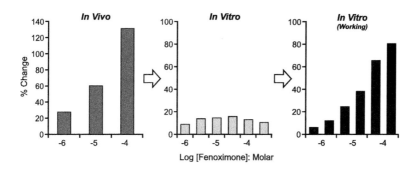

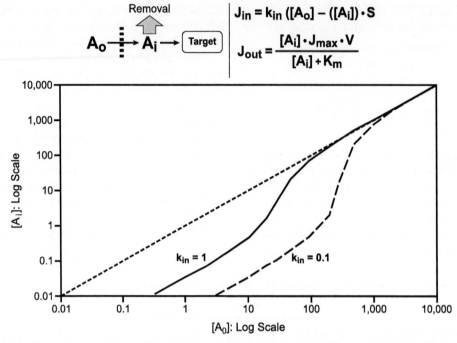

FIGURE 6.12 Drug concentration gradients under conditions of restricted diffusion. The bulk diffusion of enzyme inhibitor [A] (J_{in}) is driven by a concentration gradient and a diffusion constant k_{in}. It is assumed that the inhibitor is destroyed or otherwise diffuses out of the cell via a saturable process J_{out}. Depending on the rate of diffusion into the cell, there can be a deficit in concentration of inhibitor inside the cell ([A_i]) compared to concentrations outside the cell ([A_o]), such that [A_i]/[A_o]<1. This deficit can be overcome by high concentrations of inhibitor.

contrast, high values of $V_{max}/k_t \cdot K_m$ lead to a wide range for the dose–response curve to the enzyme inhibitor. Similarly, Fig. 6.11B shows the effect of second messenger production in cells with high enzyme activity. Again it can be seen that if basal second messenger levels are not high, there is little observed response to the enzyme inhibitor curve. These effects are important in the detection and quantitation of enzyme inhibition in cells. Box 6.5 shows how a sub-threshold level of activation of cardiac β-adreno-ceptors is required to produce direct effects of the PDE inhibitor Fenoximone; this mimics the observed *in vivo* effects of this drug where an ambient sympathetic tone (β-adenoceptor activa-tion) is present.

There can be dissimulations between the con-centration of inhibitor in the extracellular space (delivered by pharmacokinetics from the central compartment; see Chapters 7 and 8) and the actual concentration of the inhibitor at the enzyme. For example, if diffusion into the cell is slow and the clearance from the body is rapid, then the concentration in the cell available for enzyme inhibition may be chronically lower than the peak levels of drug in the plasma. Figure 6.12 shows the effect of restricted diffu-sion of an enzyme inhibitor into the cell. In the figure, [A_o] and [A_i] refer to the respective con-centrations of inhibitor outside and inside the cell. It can be seen that as the rate constant for cell entry (k_{in}) diminishes, the deficit between the inside and outside concentrations increases. While this deficit can be overcome by very high levels of inhibitor, there is a concentra-tion range whereby extracellular drug levels are

BOX 6.6

INTRACELLULAR TRANSPORT TRUMPS ENZYME ACTIVITY IN WHOLE CELL ENZYME INHIBITION

Enzyme inhibitors must enter the cell to cause effects on intracellular enzymes. The anti-cancer benzoquinazoline folate analog 1843U89 is a potent non-competitive inhibitor of thymidylate synthase ($K_i = 90$ pM). It gains access to the cell cytosol by being transported into the cell via the reduced folate carrier; the K_t for transport into human cells is 0.33 μM. While this compound is a potent inhibitor of cancer growth in human cells, it is 80- to 1300-fold less active as an anti-cancer compound in mouse. Subsequent studies have shown that 1843U89 is 80-fold less active as a substrate for transport into the cell in mouse L1210 versus human MOLT-4 cells. Thus, the inability to enter the tumor causes the striking difference in cellular activity of this compound (data from [7]).

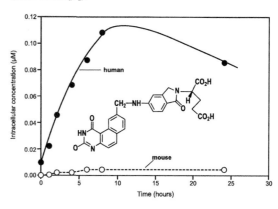

not reflected inside the cell; this would cause subsequent lower therapeutic inhibition for an intracellular enzyme. Box 6.6 gives an example of how the therapeutic effects of an anti-cancer drug are completely controlled by how well the drug can access the enzyme in the cell.

SUMMARY

- Enzymes are ubiquitous catalysts of biochemical reactions and as such furnish many potential drug targets.
- The most common therapeutic approach to enzyme control is inhibition; there are four general classes of enzyme inhibition based on the relative affinity of the inhibitor for the enzyme and the enzyme–substrate complex.
- Competitive inhibition describes inhibitors that have exclusive affinity for the enzyme and compete for substrate binding.

- Mixed inhibitors bind to the enzyme and the enzyme–substrate complex with different affinity.
- Non-competitive inhibitors bind equally well to the enzyme and enzyme–substrate complex.
- Uncompetitive inhibitors bind only to the enzyme–substrate complex.
- These different inhibitory mechanisms yield different relationships between the potency of the inhibitor and the concentration of the substrate.
- Irreversible inhibitors can also be therapeutically useful; measuring their activity requires special techniques observing the kinetics of enzyme inhibition.
- Although less common than inhibitors, enzyme activators can also be useful therapeutically.
- There are special considerations for the blockade of enzymes in cells in that concentrations may differ (from the

extracellular medium). In addition, enzyme inhibitors may have no effect until the enzyme is active metabolically under *in vivo* conditions.

QUESTIONS

6.1 A biochemical kinase assay showed that a test compound for cancer had an IC_{50} of 10 nM. In contrast, there was no significant antitumor activity found *in vivo*. What could be the issues and how could they be addressed?

6.2 ATP levels in cells can be high; therefore, competitive inhibitors of kinases can have correspondingly low potency. What would be a good type of enzyme inhibitor for this type of scenario?

6.3 The IC_{50} for a test enzyme inhibitor was found to be 30 nM when measured at 60 min and 25 nM at 120 min. In one assay, the IC_{50} was not measured until 600 min and was found to be 12 nM. Could this be indicative of a problem, and if so, why?

References

[1] M. Pal, Recent advances in glucokinase activators for the treatment of type 2 diabetes, Drug Disc. Today 14 (2009) 784–792.

[2] T.P. Kenakin, D.L. Scott, A method to assess concomitant cardiac phosphodiesterase inhibition and positive inotropy, J. Cardiovasc. Pharmacol. 10 (1987) 658–666.

[3] D.F. McGinnity, A.J. Berry, J.R. Kenny, K. Grime, R.J. Riley, Evaluation of time-dependent cytochrome P450 inhibition using cultured human hepatocytes, Drug. Metab. Dispos. 34 (2006) 1130–1291.

[4] J.A. Zorn, J.A. Wells, Turning enzymes on with small molecules, Nature Chem. Biol. 6 (2010) 179–188.

[5] D.M. Stresser, A.P. Blanchard, S.D. Turner, J.C.L. Erve, A.A. Dandeneau, V.P. Miller, et al., Substrate-dependent modulation of CYP3A4 catalytic activity: Analysis of 27 test compounds with four fluorometric substrates, Drug Metab. Dispos. 28 (2000) 1440–1448.

[6] R.C. Dage, L.E. Roebel, C.P. Hsieh, D.L. Weiner, J.K. Woodward, The effecs of MDL 17,043 on cardiac inotropy in the anaesthetized dog, J. Cardiovasc. Pharmacol. 4 (1982) 500–512.

[7] D.S. Duch, S. Banks, I.K. Dev, S.H. Dickerson, R. Ferone, L.S. Heath, et al., Biochemical and cellular pharmacology of 1843U89, a novel benzoquinazoline inhibitor of thymidylate synthase, Cancer Res. 53 (1993) 810–818.

Pharmacokinetics I: Permeation and Metabolism

By the end of this chapter the reader should appreciate how the body is a balanced *in vivo* system of inflow (absorption) and outflow (clearance) of drug, and how prospective drug molecules require a minimal set of physico-chemical properties (referred to as "drug-like") to be able to cross biological membranes to gain entry into the body. In addition, readers will learn about how passive diffusion and transport processes control absorption, while metabolism and excretion govern removal of drugs from the body. Finally, readers will see how *in vitro* metabolic assays can be used to estimate metabolic stability.

THE IMPORTANCE OF DRUG CONCENTRATION

When testing drugs *in vitro*, the drug is confined to a known volume (i.e., well of a plate,

test tube, etc.), therefore the concentration of the drug is known. This is critical since all measures of drug activity (i.e., potency, efficacy, affinity) are basically concentrations at which a defined drug effect is observed. Therefore, if a concentration of $1\,\mu M$ is seen to produce a 50% inhibition of activity, then the IC_{50} is taken to be $1\,\mu M$; this is a characteristic value that would indicate a higher potency over another drug with an IC_{50} of $10\,\mu M$ and a lower potency than one with an IC_{50} of $0.1\,\mu M$. The key to this type of system is accurate knowledge of the concentration. A useful way to view experiments is to define independent and dependent variables. Independent variables are what experimenters put into the experiment and what they are required to know; in this case, drug concentration. What comes out of an experiment is data in the form of dependent variables, i.e., what the system being observed does with the independent variable to produce a system value, i.e., potency. Independent variables have only random error whereas dependent variables have random plus system error.

In vitro data describing potency is not usually associated with a time because measurements are taken after a steady-state or equilibrium has been attained. Figure 7.1 shows the concentration of drug added to a closed vessel; the kinetics show an increase with time to a steady-state after which the dependent variable attains a constant value, i.e., it is a closed system. In contrast, *in vivo* systems are like a vessel with a hole in it; equilibrium for a single dose is not attained and the level of fluid (e.g., concentration of drug) is very much dependent on the time that the measurement is taken, i.e., they are open systems (see Fig. 7.1). Pharmacokinetics is the science of accurately determining the concentration of drug in the body and devising

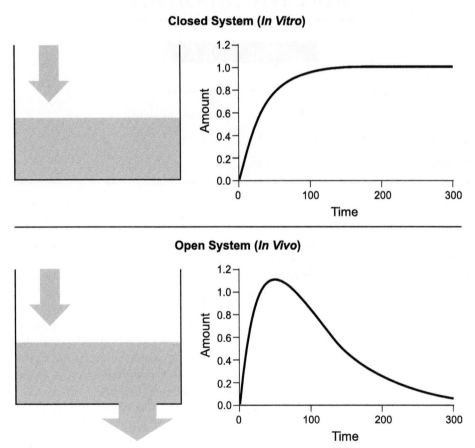

FIGURE 7.1   Model systems for drug delivery *in vitro* (top panel) and *in vivo* (bottom panel). The volume of an *in vitro* system is fixed; therefore the kinetics can be likened to filling a cup. The top right panel shows the change in fluid level with time as the vessel is filled; this level models the change in concentration of a system *in vitro* upon addition of drug. In this type of system, the concentration reaches a steady-state level. The bottom panel models an *in vivo* system where a steady-state is not attained (vessel with a hole in it). Under these circumstances, the concentration depends on the time the measurements are taken (see text).

methods of attaining steady-state levels of drug for therapy through repeat dosing. Figure 7.2 shows how giving repeated doses of a drug at regular intervals can achieve a steady-state level of drug *in vivo*. While a constant steady-state concentration of drug often can be attained *in vivo* with repeated dosing it should still be recognized that this is still a non-equilibrium system, and that the steady-state depends upon both the rate of entry and the rate of exit of the drug. Changes in either of these will subsequently alter the steady-state level of drug in the body. Figure 7.2 shows how an increase in the rate of entry of drug into the body leads to an increased steady-state, while a decrease in the rate of entry leads to a corresponding decrease in the steady-state. Figure 7.3 shows how the rate of exit of the drug correspondingly affects steady-state levels. Thus, an increased rate of exit leads to a reduced steady-state while a decrease in the rate of exit leads to an increased steady-state level. This chapter will discuss the various *in vivo* processes that control the rate of entry and exit of a drug from the body and the use of this knowledge to attain a therapeutically useful steady-state level.

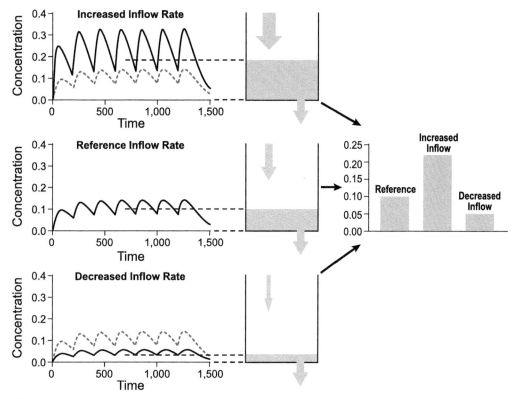

FIGURE 7.2 Repeat dosing to achieve steady-state drug levels *in vivo*. Middle panel shows how repeating a single dose of drug in an *in vivo* system can lead to a sustained level of drug after a prescribed number of doses depending on the frequency and timing of the dose (*vide infra*). The *in vivo* system is still not an equilibrium system in that it is modeled by filling a cup with a hole in it. Therefore, changes either in the rate of flow into the cup or out of the cup result in a change in the steady-state level of fluid in the cup. The top panel shows how an increase in the rate of flow into the vessel causes an increased steady-state level. The lower panel shows how a decrease in the rate of inflow causes a decrease in the steady-state level.

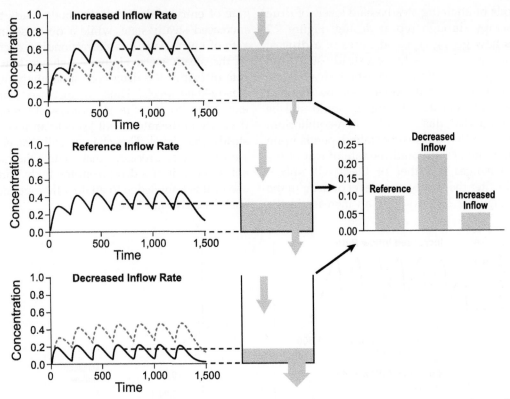

FIGURE 7.3 As shown in Fig. 7.2, repeated dosing in an *in vivo* system can lead to the attainment of a steady-state that depends on the relative rates of entry and exit from the system. The top panel shows how a decreased rate of exit can lead to an increased steady-state level while the bottom panel shows how an increase in the rate of exit leads to a decrease in the steady-state level.

Figure 7.4 shows a schematic of the various processes that affect the entry into and exit out of the body. It is worth considering these separately as a prelude to understanding how they combine to affect *in vivo* drug concentration. An acronym (ADME) is often used to describe the interaction of a molecule with these processes: absorption; distribution; metabolism and excretion. Clearly, drugs require adequate ADME properties to be therapeutically useful; Box 7.1 shows how inferior pharmacokinetics can preclude otherwise favorable *in vitro* activity.

Drugs require three basic properties: primary activity at the therapeutic target;

favorable ADME behavior to enter and stay in the body to produce effect; and a safety margin such that the drug causes no harm (Fig. 7.5). Having the correct chemical structure to confer favorable ADME properties for *in vivo* drug availability often involves separate structure–activity relationships than those required for primary therapeutic activity. The same is true for drug safety, i.e., eliminating any structural feature of the molecule that enables it to interact with a system in the body to cause harm (see Chapter 10). An illustration of how separate these structure–activity relationships can be is shown in Fig. 7.6. It can be seen from this figure that structural changes

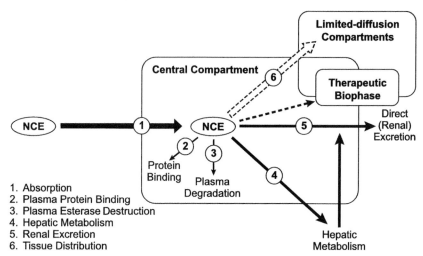

FIGURE 7.4   Schematic diagram of the various processes controlling the steady-state concentration of drug (labeled NCE for "new drug entity") introduced into the body. Measurements are made from a reference region referred to as the central compartment; this is usually the systemic circulation.

BOX 7.1

THE PRACTICAL IMPORTANCE OF PHARMACOKINETICS

Inadequate ADME properties can be devastating to otherwise good drug activity; shown below are two antitumor molecules, one five times more potent than the other. The poor pharmacokinetic properties of the more potent compound make it far less active *in vivo*.[7] Several iterations may be required before a suitable drug candidate profile is achieved. While the first histamine H2 antagonist for ulcer treatment, burimamide, had primary target activity, it required further work to develop metiamide (target active but an inadequate safety profile) and finally cimetidine (target active, safe and acceptable ADME properties) to achieve drug status. Pharmacokinetic problems led to a rate of 40% failure in drug development in 1991. Access to economical *in vitro* ADME assays led to a decrease in failure rate to 10% in 2000.[8]

$IC_{50} = 0.004$ nm   → 5-fold ↓ in potency $IC_{50} = 0.021$ nM

Very weak *in vivo* activity
Low solubility

High active *in vivo*
High solubility

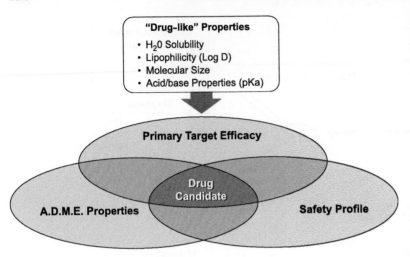

FIGURE 7.5 Four important elements of chemical structure for drugs. Overall, drugs require a set of physico-chemical properties that allow them to solubilize in aqueous media, but also to cross lipid membranes. In addition, the three main activities that a molecule needs to have to be a therapeutic entity are activity at the primary target, the pharmacokinetic properties to enter the body and be present at the target for a sufficient time to produce effect, and to not cause harm to the host. These three main activities may have different structure–activity relationships

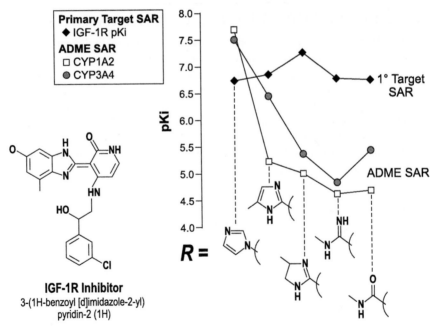

FIGURE 7.6 Analogs of an insulin growth factor receptor antagonist showing how changes in the nature of the R group lead to striking changes in the activity of the molecule at cytochrome P450 enzymes CYP1A2 and CYP3A4 (that would lead to drug–drug interactions; *vide infra*) but relatively no change in the primary IGF-1R activity. Data redrawn from [1].

that have little effect on the primary activity (in this case inhibition of insulin-like growth factor receptor-1) produce a two to three order of magnitude change in a debilitating effect on cytochrome P450 enzyme inhibiton that could cause a damaging drug–drug interaction (*vide infra*).[1]

There is a general set of physico-chemical properties common to the majority of therapeutically successful drugs; these are referred to as "drug-like" properties. Drug discovery and development common experience has shown that pro-active efforts to incorporate certain drug-like properties into prospective drug candidates greatly reduce late stage attrition in the development process (see Box 7.2). It is worth considering some of the most common drug-like activities in this light.

BOX 7.2

INTRODUCING ADME PROPERTIES: THE SOONER THE BETTER

Prior to 1990, a common practice in drug discovery was to optimize primary target activity with the idea of modifying structures for ADME activity later in the process. This can be problematic since the molecular structure may be such that any changes could lead to loss of activity, i.e., there would be insufficient places in the chemical scaffold to modify ADME properties without compromising the original activity. This is illustrated by a sample of drugs shown below, where it can be seen that the original lead molecule obtained from the screening process is extraordinarily similar to the final drug. This supports the notion of having molecules in screening libraries that already have favorable ADME properties (data from [2]).

Lead Molecule → Drug

Frovatriptan

Bulaquine

Perospirone

NEW TERMINOLOGY

The following new terms will be introduced in this chapter:

- **ADME**: Acronym for absorption, distribution, metabolism and excretion, four primary elements of pharmacokinetics.
- **Antedrug**: Molecule that is itself an active drug but is also unstable such that as it is absorbed into the body, it is metabolized to an inactive compound.
- **Bioavailability**: This parameter quantifies the amount of drug that is available for physiological action in the central compartment after absorption.
- **Central compartment**: The main circulation (bloodstream) from where pharmacokinetic sampling of drug levels is taken.
- **Clearance**: The removal of drug from the body in units of volume per unit time (e.g., mL min $^{-1}$).
- **Dependent variable**: Experimental observation taken from a system that has taken an independent variable and yielded a system response.
- **Drug−drug interaction**: When one drug interferes with the pharmacokinetics of another drug in the body to produce an adverse effect.
- **Drug-like**: The physico-chemical properties of molecules that cause them to be successful drugs *in vivo*.
- **Enzyme induction**: The reaction of the liver to pharmacokinetic stress such that levels of metabolic enzyme activity increase either through activation of gene expression, stabilization of mRNA or PXR activation.
- **First pass effect**: The metabolic gauntlet for drugs taken orally whereby they must first be absorbed through the gastrointestinal lumen and then immediately pass through the liver via the portal vein to be metabolized.

- **Independent variable**: The experimental quantity (usually drug dose or concentration) known by the experimenter that is processed by the system to yield the dependent variable.
- *In vitro* **system**: Latin for "within the glass," this term refers to an experiment done in a controlled environment. For pharmacology it is when experiments are done in contained vessels and where concentration is known (a closed system).
- *In vivo* **system**: "Within a living organism," this term refers to experiments done in the whole body (an open system).
- **Lipophilicity**: The ability of a molecule to dissolve in lipids or organic solvents such as octanol or heptane, as opposed to water.
- **LogP (LogD)**: Logarithm of the ratio of the solubility of a compound in organic medium versus aqueous medium. cLogP is calculated and mLogP is measured. Log D takes into account ionized species in the aqueous medium and must be reported with a distinct pH value.
- **MAD**: "Maximal absorbable dose" is the maximum amount of drug that can be expected to be absorbed from the GI tract when a compound is given orally.
- **Mechanism-based inhibition (also time-dependent inhibition)**: Blockade of an enzyme that is essentially irreversible. The onset time for full blockade is prolonged and new enzyme activity can only be obtained through synthesis of new enzyme.
- **PAMPA**: "Parallel artificial membrane permeation assay" consisting of a synthetic hexadecane lipid membrane layered over a screen to allow measurement of molecules traversing the membrane via bulk lipid diffusion.
- **Permeation (P_{app})**: The rate of transfer of a molecule across a membrane (usually expressed in cm s $^{-1}$).
- **pK_a**: Negative logarithm of equilibrium equation describing relative amounts of a

molecule in the acid/base form over the unionized form.

- **Prodrug**: Molecule that itself is not biologically active but is optimized to be absorbed into the body. Once the molecule is absorbed, biological or chemical processes transform the prodrug into the active drug.
- $t_{\frac{1}{2}}$: The time required for the amount of substance, decaying as a result of an exponential process, to decrease to half of its initial value.

"DRUG-LIKE" PROPERTIES OF MOLECULES

The physico-chemical properties of molecules that are important to their function as drugs can be summarized under the following headings:

1. Water solubility;
2. Lipophilicity;
3. pK_A and acid/base properties;
4. molecular weight.

It is worth considering these separately.

1. **Water solubility**: A molecule *must* dissolve in water before it can interact with any process in the body, including passage through lipid membranes. Molecules can have a wide range of solubility in water and this can greatly affect how well they are absorbed and metabolized, how they distribute through the body compartments and how they are excreted. An indication of how important water solubility is can be determined from consideration of MAD (maximal absorbable dose) values. This is basically the maximal amount of drug that can be absorbed orally if the small intestine (the site for oral drug absorption) were saturated with the drug (i.e., the maximum amount dissolved in water) for 4.5 hours (the

transit time for intestinal contents). The MAD is given by:

$$MAD = S \times Kab \times SIWV \times SITT \quad (7.1)$$

where: S is H_2O solubility in mg ml^{-1} at pH 6.5, K_{ab} is the transintestinal absorption rate constant (min^{-1}), SIWV is the small intestine water volume ($\approx$250 mL) and SITT is the small intestine transit time ($\approx$4.5 hours). Calculation of the MAD can be revealing. For example, if a required therapeutic level of a drug were 0.5 mg kg^{-1}, then 35 mg would need to be absorbed for a 70 kg patient. If a given drug has an absorption rate constant from the intestine of 0.03 min^{-1} and a low solubility (0.001 mg mL^{-1}), the MAD would only be 2 mg, well below that needed for any effect. For cases of low absorption, solubility may be much more amenable to change than intestinal absorption. The latter value generally can effectively be increased by a factor of 50 (from 0.001 to 0.05 min^{-1}) through medicinal chemistry, whereas solubility can change by five orders of magnitude (0.001 to 100 mg mL^{-1}). In the previous example, chemical modification to increase water solubility to a value of 0.02 mg mL^{-1} would put the drug in the therapeutic range (MAD = 40 mg). A high water solubility for a drug molecule is 85% solubility at pH values from 1 to 7.5 occurring in less than 30 minutes.

2. **Lipophilicity**: This is the degree to which the drug molecule will dissolve in organic media; it is a surrogate for how well the drug will dissolve in biological lipid membranes. This can be estimated through LogP or LogD values which can, in turn, be measured or calculated through indices associated with chemical groups on the molecule. LogP values are logarithms of the relative concentration of the molecule dissolved in an organic medium such as octanol or heptane versus that dissolved in water. Thus, a LogP value of 0.5 indicates a fairly water-soluble molecule with a ratio of

3.16 to 1 for octanol to water. LogP values >3 indicate highly lipid-soluble molecules (ratio octanol to water of >1000 to 1). LogD values are the same as LogP values except, unlike the latter, they also include the ionic species. For this reason they must be reported with a given pH value, as the ionization of molecules can change at different pH values (*vide infra*). The dependence of cellular absorption on LogP or LogD values illustrates the particular dichotomous behavior drug molecules must have toward aqueous and organic media, i.e., drugs must dissolve in water but also in lipid to interact with biological systems and cross membranes; this will be considered further in discussion of drug absorption. A drug-like value for LogP ranges from 0.5 < LogP < 3. LogP and Log D values are widely used in the structure–activity analyses of ADME properties, since they are readily available for molecules and can be correlated with a wide range of ADME processes. Of a sample of 1791 approved drugs, the mean LogP value is 2.5.[2]

3. **Acid/base properties**: Molecules can function as acids or bases in aqueous media depending on the ability of various chemical groups to lose or gain hydrogen ions. The ease with which this occurs depends on the pH of the medium. The relationship between the propensity of a molecule to be in an acidic or basic state and the pH is given by the Henderson–Hasslebach equation:

$$pKa = pH + Log([acid\ form]/[base\ form])$$

(7.2)

where pK_a refers to the $-$logarithm of the K_a which is a dissociation constant of a molecular species HB such that $K_a = [H^+][B]/[HB]$ (B is the conjugate base of the molecule HB). The important point to note is that the pK_a of a given molecule can dictate the relative amount of ionic species in the aqueous medium. Since ions do not cross lipid barriers through bulk diffusion, this can affect drug absorption. For example, the decongestant phenylpropanolamine has a pK_a of 9.4 which indicates that it essentially exists in the charged conjugate acid form throughout all of the physiological range of pH (1.5 to 7.8). The population of known drugs has a huge range of pK_a from 1 (dapsone) to nearly 14 (caffeine). The pK_a is mainly used to assess drug absorption and distribution in pharmacokinetic studies.

4. **Molecular weight**: Extremely large molecules do not cross plasma–lipid membranes well; therefore a molecular weight <350 is a good target for drug-like activity. Of a sample of all marketed drugs up to 1995, the median molecular weight is 350. However, there are classes of drug that seem to require greater mass, e.g., HIV protease and renin inhibitors have a median molecular weight of 680–700.

In general, the physico-chemical properties of a molecule should be within certain ranges for drug-like activity but exceptions to these rules can be found in every category (see Box 7.3). A frequently used guideline is the so-called "rule of 5" reported by Lipinski and colleagues.[3,4] From an analysis of 2245 drug-like compounds, it was observed that 89% had a molecular weight <550, only 10% had a calculated LogP >5.0, only 8% had a sum of OH and NH (hydrogen bond donors) groups >5 and only 12% had the sum of N and O atoms (hydrogen bond acceptors) >10. From these facts came a set of four rules involving the number 5 suggesting that poor absorption or permeation would be more likely from molecules that had:

- >5 H-bond donors;
- >10 hydrogen bond acceptors;
- >500 molecular weight;
- >5 calculated LogP.

Once a molecule that has been synthesized shows primary therapeutic target activity in

BOX 7.3

WATER VERSUS LIPID SOLUBILITY OF DRUGS

Guidelines for drug absorption can be derived from solubility and LogP data, but there are exceptions. For instance, azithromycin has an extremely low transintestinal absorption rate constant ($K_{ab} = 0.001$ min^{-1}) normally predictive of very poor absorption. However, the extraordinarily high solubility of this molecule (>50 mg mL^{-1}) allows it to have a very high MAD of 3.75 g.[9]

Usually, exceedingly high LogP values are associated with lack of membrane permeation due to the fact that the molecules may lodge in the lipid membrane and not traverse the cell (i.e., dihydropyridines). High LogP values are also associated with non-specific activity and undesirable drug profiles. However, torcetrapib, a drug for dyslipidemia targeting cholesterol ester transfer protein, has a cLogP of 8.2. In this case, the natural substrates for this target are cholesterol esters (cLogP = 18) thus the high LogP for torcetrapib is a requirement for activity.[10]

the appropriate *in vitro* systems and does not greatly violate drug-like property rules, it can be tested *in vivo*; under these conditions it must enter the human body to reach the therapeutic target organ and remain in the target compartment long enough to produce therapeutic activity. The first step in this process is absorption.

DRUG ABSORPTION

All drugs must cross cell lipid bilayer membranes to reach their site of action in the body. The rate at which they do this, coupled with the rate at which they are removed from the compartment into which they diffuse, dictates the overall concentration in the compartment (as shown in Figs 7.2 and 7.3). One of the most important mechanisms to enable passage through membranes is bulk diffusion. Figure 7.7 shows three possible outcomes for a molecule interacting with a cell membrane; the molecule may or may not pass through the membrane or it may dissolve and stay in the membrane. The relative propensity of the molecule to dissolve in water and lipid dictates which of these will occur; as discussed previously, a useful measure of water to lipid solubility is the LogP or LogD value for the

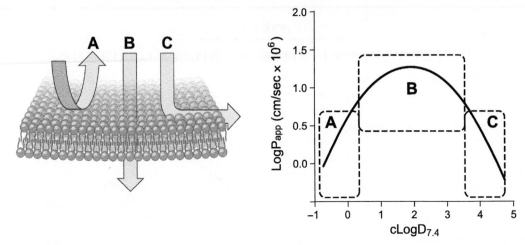

FIGURE 7.7 Diffusion through lipid membranes. Region A contains compounds of low LogP values (highly water-soluble). These may not penetrate lipid membranes and remain in the aqueous phase. Region B contains molecules that dissolve both in water and lipid (0.5 < LogP < 3.0) and thus may cross lipid membranes. Highly lipid-soluble compounds (region C; LogP > 3) may dissolve in the membrane and not emerge (i.e., dihydropyridines). Graph on right shows the relationship between permeation and cLogD$_{7.4}$

molecule. If a molecule is highly soluble in water (LogP $\leq$ 0.5) it will not penetrate lipid membranes well (Fig. 7.7 region A). A molecule with solubility both in water and lipid (0.5 < LogP < 3.0; Fig. 7.7 region B) may cross lipid membranes while an extremely lipid-soluble molecule (LogP > 3) may dissolve in the lipid membrane and stay there (Fig 7.7 region C). Bulk diffusion is driven by a concentration gradient, thus there will be a flow of molecules from the region of high concentration (i.e., outside the cell) to a region of low concentration (inside the cell and/or beyond the cell layer barrier). A system has been devised that considers how well molecules permeate lipid membranes and also their water solubility. Termed the BCS system, it generally predicts how well molecules will be absorbed (see Box 7.4).

In addition to bulk diffusion, cells may cross cell membranes through a transport process such as:

- **Facillitated diffusion**: An oscillating carrier protein shuttles molecules across the membrane. These processes are concentration-gradient driven and do not require energy. They generally transport sugars and other nutrients and are not especially relevant to drugs.
- **Active transport**: Passage across the membrane is mediated by a saturable transport process that requires energy. These can operate against a concentration gradient and are important in the liver, kidney, gut epithelium and blood−brain barrier (*vide infra*). Importantly, they can operate to take molecules both inside and outside of the cell.

Figure 7.8 shows three important mechanisms for molecular transfer across cell lipid membranes; bulk diffusion, transport into the cell (influx) and transport out of the cell (efflux). In many cases, all three of these may be operable for drug entry into the cell and beyond a cellular barrier such as the intestinal tract. It is important to note that, since the transport processes are saturable and bulk diffusion is not, the overall rate of uptake of a molecule into the cell can be concentration-dependent. This

BOX 7.4

THE BIOPHARMACEUTICS CLASSIFICATION SYSTEM (BCS)

The BCS system ranks molecules in terms of solubility and permeability. For Class 1 molecules (ideal for oral drugs) the rate of dissolution limits absorption. Class 2 molecules typically require formulation since solubility limits absorption. For Class 3 molecules, permeability limits absorption; in these cases a prodrug strategy is often employed. While LogP values can be useful guidelines for solubility, wide variations can be observed. For example, in spite of a 21,000-fold difference in LogP values for clazozimine (LogP = 5.39) and levonorgestrel (LogP = 0.06), they have equal water solubilities (0.01 mg mL^{-1}). [11]

	High Solubility	Low Solubility
High Permeability	**Class 1 (amphiphilic)** Nortriptylene Diltiazem Captopril Labetolol Enalapril Propranolol Metoprolol	**Class 2 (lipophilic)** Phenytoin Diclofenac Naproxen Piroxicam Carbamazepine Flurbiprofen
Low Permeability	**Class 3 (hydrophilic)** Cimetidine Atenolol Ranitidine Nadolol Femotidine	**Class 4** Hydrochlorthiazide Furosemide Ketoprofen Terfenadine

means that, depending on where the process is being viewed (i.e., GI tract versus therapeutic cell in the central compartment), diffusion, influx and efflux can be of varying importance. Efflux processes (such as P-gp, p-Glycoprotein transport) shuttle molecules that have already entered the cell and transport them out of the cell again; they are designed to protect cells from foreign chemicals. As shown in Fig. 7.8, an efflux process can effectively stop entry into the cell at low concentrations (see curve for observed absorption). However, if the molecule diffuses through lipid membranes, then high concentrations that saturate the efflux process can still enter cells. Similarly, if a drug is transported into the cell, then lower doses may rely more on this mechanism than on bulk diffusion. This may be important for low concentrations of drug that are transported into hepatic cells for degradation.

On a more general note, molecules must not only enter cells but must cross into and back out of cells in a vectorial manner to gain access to therapeutically relevant compartments in

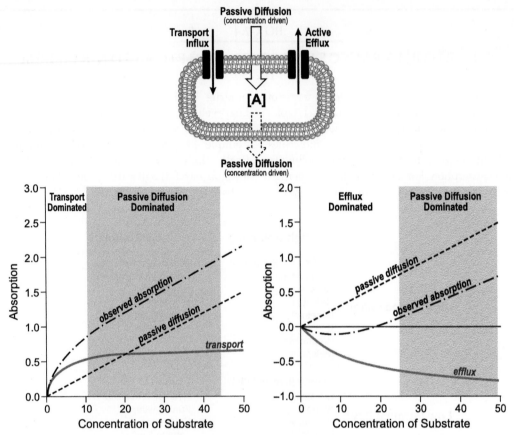

FIGURE 7.8 Mechanisms of entry into and through cells. Molecule A may enter the cell through bulk diffusion through the lipid membrane and/or an influx through a transport carrier. It can leave the cell through bulk diffusion (although this is concentration driven and thus the flow will be to the region of lower concentration) or an efflux carrier. The efflux carrier can proceed against a concentration gradient, thus it serves as a barrier to absorption while diffusion promotes absorption. Influx and efflux mechanisms are saturable with respect to concentration (curved Michaelis–Menten-like curves) while diffusion is not (straight line). Bottom panels show how overall transfer of molecules through cells is the sum of diffusion and influx–efflux. It can be seen that low concentrations are more subject to transport processes, making overall entry dependent on concentration. It can also be seen that low concentrations may be dominated by efflux processes, but that these can be overcome through bulk diffusion of higher concentrations.

the body. A useful model of this larger scale absorption is the transfer of molecules from the lumen of the GI tract to the bloodstream. Figure 7.9 shows a range of processes operative when cells cross the GI epithelial cell layer to gain access to the central compartment. In addition to bulk diffusion and influx, and battling efflux processes, molecules may be destroyed by metabolic enzymes as they try to cross the epithelial cell layer. Notably, the metabolic enzyme cytochrome P450 type 3A4, an extremely common metabolizing enzyme for drug molecules (*vide infra*), is present in these cells and can notably deplete the concentration of drug as it passes from the lumen into the bloodstream. The most formidable

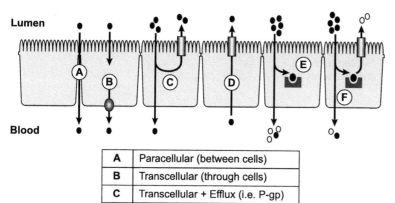

FIGURE 7.9 Processes operative as molecules cross cell layers to gain access to the central compartment through epithelial cells from the lumen of the gastrointestinal tract. (A) Molecules may pass through small openings between cells (8 to 10 angstroms); (B) cross the cell membrane through bulk diffusion or an influx transport process or both; (C) cross through membranes via diffusion and influx but are also subject to apical efflux (i.e., P-gp); (D) bulk diffusion can also cause reverse passage of drug from the central compartment to lumen (minor); (E) molecules enter the cell but then are metabolized and (F) molecules enter the cell, are metabolized and also are removed from the cell through active efflux.

A	Paracellular (between cells)
B	Transcellular (through cells)
C	Transcellular + Efflux (i.e. P-gp)
D	Apical Efflux
E	Intracellular Metabolism
F	Intracellular Metabolism + Efflux

barrier to lumen–bloodstream absorption is a combination of metabolic degradation and active efflux from the cell (process F in Fig. 7.9).

There are very useful *in vitro* model systems that can be used to measure the ability of molecules to pass through membranes (measured as permeation values (P_{app}) with units of rate $\times 10^{-5}$ cm s^{-1}). For passive lipid membrane diffusion, the rate of passage through a phospholipid coated filter membrane (referred to as PAMPA for Parallel Artificial Membrane Permeation Assay) is measured. Permeation through biological membranes can also be measured *in vitro* by passing molecules through a layer of cells designed to model the gastrointestinal tract. The most commonly used cells are CacCo-2 cells (human colonic adrenocarcinoma cells). These preparations allow molecules to pass through the lipid membrane by bulk diffusion as well as through influx transport and also to encounter efflux transport processes such as P-gp. Comparison of permeation values in PAMPA and Caco-2 assays can be used to determine whether molecules primarily cross membranes through bulk diffusion or if they are substrates

of either active influx or active efflux processes (see Fig. 7.10). Similarly, the bidirectional permeation across CaCo-2 cells can be used to detect efflux mechanisms such as P-gp. In this case, the P_{app} for transfer from the basal to the apical side (inside to outside) will be greater than P_{app} values for diffusion from the apical to the basal side (outside to inside). If this difference is eliminated by efflux transporter inhibitors (such as verapamil for P-gp) then activity of an efflux transporter is confirmed. While CaCo-2 cells have proven extremely serviceable in ADME permeation studies, there are exceptions to their predictive value. For example β-Lactam antibiotics (cephalexin, amoxicillin) and ACE inhibitors are good substrates for peptide transporters and have poor permeability in Caco-2 cells, yet these drugs are completely absorbed *in vivo* in humans.

Drug absorption is important for the entry of molecules into cells for therapy and also for entry into the body, especially via the oral route of administration. This latter important process is greatly affected by drug metabolism so it will be considered later in this chapter after metabolism has been discussed. At this

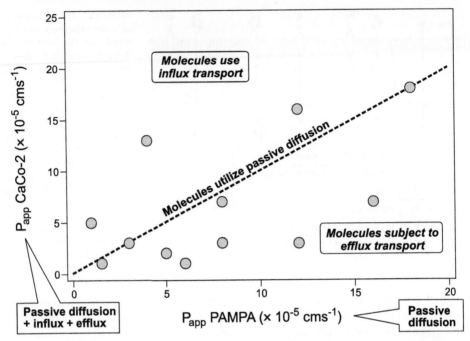

FIGURE 7.10　Difference in permeation values for compounds in a passive diffusion assay (abscissa) and a biological membrane assay (ordinates). If P_{app} values are the same in each assay, then the presence of influx or efflux does not alter permeation, supporting the view that passive diffusion is the primary mechanism. If P_{app} in PAMPA is greater than CaCo-2, then a retarding efflux in the biological membrane is suggested. Similarly, if P_{app} in CaCo-1 is greater than PAMPA, then the presence of an assisting influx transporter in the biological membrane is suggested.

time it is also worth considering other methods of introducing drugs into the body. Table 7.1 shows the various common routes of drug administration and some of their salient features. With the exception of parenteral administration directly into the bloodstream, absorption is an important element of available drug levels.

There are certain physico-chemical molecular properties that are important for drug absorption (correct LogP, molecular size, etc.) and there are some situations where the structure−activity relationships required for primary drug activity cannot be reconciled with those required for absorption. Under these circumstances, a prodrug of the active drug molecule may need to be used *in vivo*. A prodrug

is a metabolically unstable derivative of the active drug that is itself well absorbed but degrades to the active drug in the central compartment after absorption (see Fig. 7.11 and Box 7.5). Some commonly used drugs that actually are administered as prodrugs are Enalapril (esterase release of active moiety enalaprilat for hypertension), Valaciclovir (esterase release of acyclovir for herpes) and Levodopa (DOPA decarboxylase-mediated release of dopamine for Parkinson's disease). A variation of this theme is an antedrug which is a molecule that has limited distribution and absorption properties due to the fact that it degrades to a non-absorbable and/or inactive derivative after leaving the active therapeutic compartment (Fig 7.11).

TABLE 7.1 Routes of Administration for Drugs

Route	Advantages	Disadvantages
PARENTERAL		
Intravenous	• rapid attainment of concentration • precise delivery of dosage • easy to titrate dose	• high initial concentration: toxicity • invasive: risk of infection • requires skill
Subcutaneous	• prompt absorption from aqueous • little training needed • avoid harsh GI environment • can be used for suspensions	• cannot be used for large volumes • potential pain/tissue damage • variable absorption
ENTERAL		
Oral	• convenient (storage/portability) • economical/non-invasive/safe • requires no training	• delivery can be erratic • depends on patient compliance • drugs degrade in GI environment • first pass effect
Sublingual	• rapid onset • avoids first pass	• few drugs adequately absorbed • patients must avoid swallowing • difficult compliance
Pulmonary	• easy to titrate dose/rapid onset • local effect/minimizes toxic effects	• requires coordination • lung disease limits • variable delivery
Topical	• minimize side-effects • avoids first pass effect	• cosmetically unappealing • erratic absorption

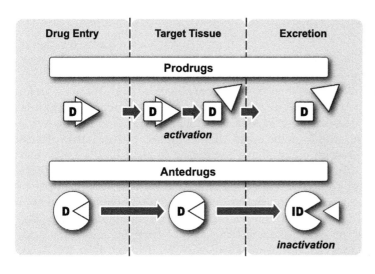

FIGURE 7.11 Two strategies for controlling drug absorption. *Prodrugs* are derivatives of an active drug that are well absorbed. Once in the therapeutic compartment they are degraded to the active drug. *Antedrugs* are unstable active drugs that reach the therapeutic compartment and are then degraded to inactive products before they distribute further in the body.

BOX 7.5

PRODRUGS: STRATEGIES FOR DRUG DELIVERY

There are cases where a valuable drug therapy cannot be delivered to the organ where it is required. Also, there are some compartments of the body that have restricted access (i.e., cerebrospinal, endolymph, synovial, pleural fluid). One of these is the eye which, in addition to providing an aqueous outward flow that prevents entry, also requires drugs to cross the cornea. A useful molecule to lower the elevated pressure in the eye in glaucoma is the natural hormone epinephrine. However, this molecule does not cross the cornea, making administration of epinephrine in glaucoma a problem. The diester dipivalylepinephrine crosses the cornea readily and when this molecule enters the eye, esterases release the active epinephrine molecule. Prodrugs can also be used to limit side-effects, a strategy often used for drugs administered by aerosol in the lung, where the surface area for absorption in humans is the size of a tennis court. This method of delivery is rapid, avoids first pass degradation in the liver, presents the drug in a high concentration at the organ for treatment (i.e., bronchioles) and then diffuses in much lower concentrations at organs where safety may be an issue (i.e., the heart).

DRUG METABOLISM

Foreign chemicals are destroyed by metabolic enzymes present in numerous regions of the body including the lungs, intestinal and nasal mucosa, brain, plasma, kidney and the liver. In general, however, the most important organ in the body for protection from foreign chemicals is the liver. This organ directly receives chemicals ingested by the oral route and acts as a cyclic filter of chemicals introduced by other means (parenterally, topically or via aerosol). It is designed to destroy all chemicals foreign to the body and does so through an extensive collection of degradative enzymes. There are two general classes of metabolic reactions present in the liver known as Phase 1 (functionalization) and Phase 2 (conjugation) reactions. Phase 1 reactions introduce or expose functional groups into the molecule which can then be linked to functional groups by Phase 2 enzymes to yield highly polar (and usually inactive) metabolites that are rapidly excreted by the renal system. An example of this process for the drug Phenytoin is shown in Fig. 7.12. Phase 1 reactions are mainly carried out by a class of enzymes known as cytochrome P450s (CYPs). The 63 gene family of

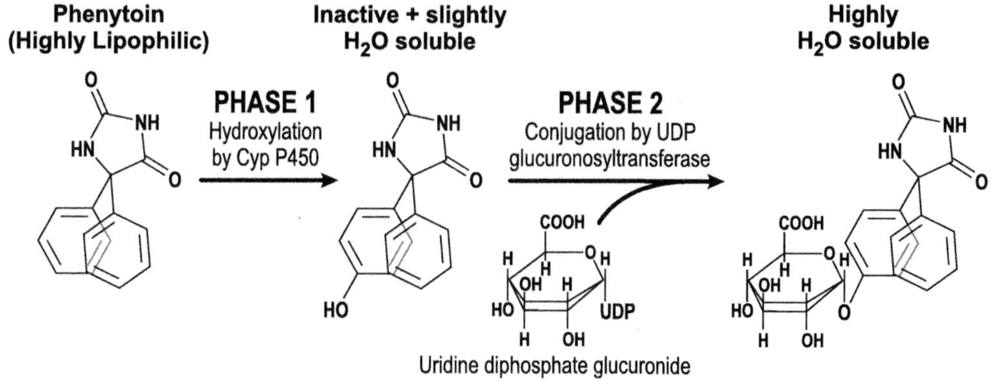

FIGURE 7.12 The metabolism of Phenytoin, an anticonvulsant used for the treatment of seizures. Phase 1 hydroxylation converts the lipophilic active drug into a more water-soluble inactive hydroxylated product which then undergoes Phase 2 metabolism to a highly soluble and readily excretable product through conjugation with uridine diphosphate glucuronide.

cytochrome P450 enzymes makes up the bulk of the metabolizing function of the liver. They are membrane-bound enzymes in the endoplasmic reticulum that have an amazing diversity in the types of substrates they can attack (see Box 7.6); they generally insert a molecule of oxygen into their substrates. There are a number of possible outcomes for these reactions:

- Active drug → inactive metabolite (most common); e.g., hydroxylation of phenobarbital to hydroxyphenobarbital.
- Active drug → active metabolite; e.g., acetylation of procainamide to N-acetylprocainamide.
- Inactive drug → active metabolite; e.g., demethylation of codeine to morphine.
- Active drug → reactive metabolite; e.g., acetaminophen → reactive metabolite.

Of the choices above, the formation of reactive metabolites is the most damaging since this can produce lasting harm to the body (*vide infra*).

Hepatic enzymes (notably cytochrome P450 enzymes) are numerous and the liver has them in variable quantities that may adjust in accordance with the metabolic stress experienced by the organ. In practical terms, there are certain main CYPs that do much of the metabolizing of most drugs. Thus, the most prevalent forms of CYPs in the human liver are CYP3A4/5/7, CYP2D6, CYP2C8/9/18, CYP3E1, CYP2A6 and CYP1A1/2. Approximately 80% of known drugs are metabolized by CYP3A4, CYP2D6, CYP2C19, CYP2A6, CYP2E1, CYP1A2 and CYP2C8–10. Some of these are more variable (both in quantity and genetics) than others and this can lead to more pharmacokinetic variability in drug studies for the drugs involved. For example, in random samples of human liver, there can be a variation of over 500-fold in the quantity of CYP2D6. In addition, there can be considerable genetic variability leading to functional polymorphism (notably for CYP2A6, CYP2C9, CYP2C19 and CYP2D6). For example, polymorphisms in CYP2C19 affect 20% of all Asians and 3% of Caucasians, leading to Japanese/Chinese susceptibility to ethanol effects.

Before further discussion of drug metabolism, it is important to consider the form of the drug being metabolized once it enters the central compartment. Once the drug enters the

BOX 7.6

THE AMAZING RANGE OF CYP3A4

Most enzymes are optimized for a given substrate to preserve the fidelity of cellular signaling. Cytochrome P450s, however, have a huge range of possible substrates to best equip them to metabolize diverse foreign chemicals. Below are a few of the known substrates for CYP3A4. Circles denote site of CYP3A4 metabolism.

general circulation, there are processes that can compromise free drug concentration. One of the most important of these is plasma protein binding. Human plasma contains more than 60 proteins, some of which can bind small drug molecules. These proteins are of three general types: albumin (binding anionic drugs); α1-acid glycoprotein (binding cationic drugs) and lipoproteins. Plasma protein binding can function as a buffer between the drug and physiological processes. Thus, protein-bound drug cannot be metabolized by the hepatic system, be functionally active at the target site for therapy or be filtered by the glomerulous of the kidney to take part in renal clearance. Plasma protein binding is relevant to this section on metabolism because protein-bound drug cannot be metabolized. Therefore, when considering the concentration of drug that can be metabolized, a fraction f_u is used which simply denotes the fraction not bound by plasma protein.

Figure 7.13 shows some possible outcomes of hepatic metabolism of a molecule. In contrast to the production of an inactive metabolite, a metabolic creation of active molecule can lead to complications. In some cases, the effect could be beneficial and the parent drug may take on the role of a prodrug. This may assist in the duration of action and therapeutic utility. If the rate of formation of the metabolite is rate limiting and the metabolite has a rate of clearance greater than the parent, then the pharmacokinetics of the parent are of particular importance. If, however, the rate of clearance of a metabolite is lower than that of the parent, then separate pharmacokinetic consideration of the metabolite must be taken *in vivo*. For example hydroxyhexamide, the active metabolite of the antidiabetic drug acetohexamide, has a much slower rate of clearance than the parent. Repeat dosing with acetohexamide thus can cause accumulation of hydroxyhexamide unless the activity of this secondary molecule is considered in the dosing regimen of the parent.[5]

Hepatic metabolism also has the capability of producing a reactive molecule, i.e., a molecule that can chemically react with proteins and/or DNA to cause irreversible modification. These effects can lead to mutagenesis and cyto- and immunotoxicity. For example, the production of procarcinogens has been observed from the action of CYP1A1 on polycyclic aromatic hydrocarbons, CYP1A2 on heteropolycyclic amines, CYP3E1 on chloroform and methylene chloride, and CYP3A4 on estradiol and aflatoxin B1. The production of reactive chemical groups such as epoxides and nitrenium ions can lead to these effects as well. If this is encountered in a discovery or development program, it must be addressed chemically as it is unacceptable in a drug candidate profile.

Phase 2 reactions generally add a highly water-soluble group onto a hydroxyl (or other suitable) group on the molecule (see Fig. 7.12). Thus, conjugates can be made with glucuronic acid, sulfonates, glutathione and amino acids in reactions resulting in glucuronidation, sulfation, methylation, acetylation and mercapture formation. While Phase 2 reactions generally precede Phase 1 reactions, there are exceptions to this rule.

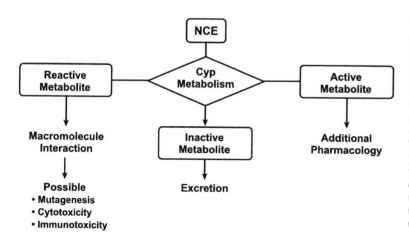

FIGURE 7.13 Possible outcomes of hepatic metabolism. A molecule could be subjected to Phase 1 metabolism to produce an inactive metabolite which then may be excreted at that point or further converted through Phase 2 metabolism to a more polar metabolite to be subsequently excreted by the renal system. This process could also yield a pharmacologically active metabolite which could produce responses in its own right. Finally, a chemically reactive metabolite may be made which then irreversibly interacts with proteins and/or DNA to produce toxicity or mutagenicity.

It is clear that hepatic degradation can be a major obstacle to attaining a stable steady-state drug concentration in the body for therapeutic use. Because of this, molecules are tested *in vitro* in hepatic enzyme preparations at an early stage of drug development to identify possible problematic chemical scaffolds. There are three major *in vitro* preparations of human liver enzymes utilized for this; microsomes, S9 fraction and hepatocytes. Liver microsomes are homogenized liver fragments partially purified through centrifugation. They can be prepared in large quantities and frozen, leading to a convenient and stable assay system. Microsomes primarily contain Phase 1 enzyme activity. Test molecules are incubated with microsomes *in vitro* and the half time ($t_{1/2}$) for disappearance of compound is used to estimate the stability of the compound in the assay. The $t_{1/2}$ is the time required for the concentration of parent to be reduced to $1/2$ of its value. For example, if one compound has a $t_{1/2}$ of 35 minutes and another of 5 minutes, then it is clear that the second compound is much less stable in the microsome preparation, i.e., it is a better substrate for Phase 1 metabolic reactions. If it is assumed that the disappearance of the compounds can be estimated by a first order decay, then a single timepoint can be used as a measure of stability. Figure 7.14 shows the degradation of a set of compounds in a microsome assay with an arrow near the percentage of compound remaining at 60 minutes. This single value then represents the stability of the compounds, i.e., a compound with 80% remaining after 60 minutes is more stable (and a poorer substrate for Phase 1 reactions) than a compound with a value of 15% remaining at 60 minutes. If the quantity of enzyme is known for the assay, then the data can be scaled to predict *in vivo* removal of compound by hepatic degradation. This is

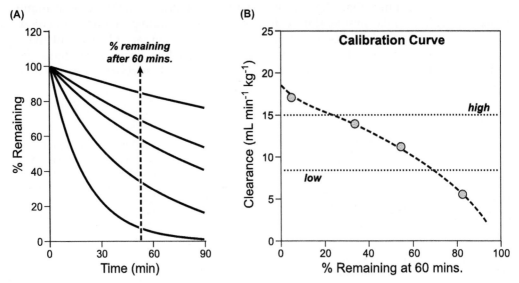

FIGURE 7.14 Estimation of compound stability in liver microsomes. (A) Degradation of a series of compounds in a microsomal assay; five compounds of varying stability are shown. A measure of stability can be obtained from a single value of percentage of parent compound remaining after 60 minutes in the assay. A select range of compounds can be studied in detail to obtain predicted clearance values from values of the percentage of remaining parent. This can furnish a calibration curve (shown in panel (B)). With this curve, large numbers of compounds can be assessed for stability at 60 minutes to estimate clearance.

termed "clearance" and it is one of the most important parameters in pharmacokinetics. It will be specifically discussed in a future section of this chapter, but for the purposes of this present discussion it is used to extrapolate the *in vitro* stability of the compound to what might be expected to be a clinical parameter *in vivo*. Thus, an unstable compound would be predicted to have a high clearance (high rate of removal) and a stable compound a lower clearance. These correlations are not absolute as the *in vitro* microsome assay gives a partial answer, i.e., Phase 2 metabolism, transport into the hepatic cell, protein binding and clearance by other routes, i.e., renal, are not considered. However, as an early indicator of pharmacokinetic problems, microsomes give a reasonable prediction of possible problems to come later in drug testing. Figure 7.14B shows a calibration curve of scaled values relating the percentage of compound remaining in the microsome assay and the predicted *in vivo* clearance. Once this is in place, the stability of hundreds of compounds can be tested at a given timepoint for a rapid estimate of predicted clearance.

In general, microsomes form the first line of hepatic *in vitro* testing. However, there are two other *in vitro* hepatic preparations used for the analysis described above. An assay utilizing a differentially centrifuged sample of microsomes termed the S9 fraction contains some Phase 2 enzymes and yields more information. Another assay utilizes hepatocytes. These are liver cells that contain the natural ratio of Phase 1 to Phase 2 enzymes and also have the added property of having the physiological transport systems (both into and out of the cell) in place to govern access of the compound to the hepatic system. While more physiological, this assay is somewhat more complex and is not as robust as microsomes or S9. In addition, it can be argued that most new drug entities do not have the functional groups required for Phase 2 metabolism (Phase 1

processes put them there) and that Phase 1 metabolism is usually rate limiting and the more important process. There can be dissimulations between data obtained from microsomes versus hepatocytes relating to access of the compounds to the enzymes. Specifically, microsomes may underestimate stability by exposing the compounds to enzymes they may never see *in vivo* (if they are not substrates of the transport process that pump them into the liver cell). Alternatively, they may overestimate stability of a compound that is actively pumped into the liver cell and thus is at a lower concentration in microsomal preparations. In any case, the scaling procedure described for microsomes above which relates *in vitro* stability to clearance can still be undertaken. Once the compound stability is determined in a mixture of CYPs, the responsible enzymes can be identified through the use of specific inhibitors; a list of common inhibitors of various CYPs is shown in Table 7.2. As an example, if $5\,\mu M$ of Furylline blocks a microsomal degradation of a given compound, this would suggest that CYP1A2 is involved.

TABLE 7.2 Some Common Inhibitors of Cytochrome P450 Enzymes

CYP	Inhibitor	Ki (μM)
1A2	Furylline	0.6−0.73
2A6	Tranylcypromine	0.02−0.2
	Methoxsalen	0.01−0.2
2B6	Sertraline	3.2
	Clopidogrel	0.5
2C8	Quercetin	1.1
2C9	Sulfaphenazole	0.3
2C19	Ticlopidine	1.2
2D6	Quinadine	0.027−0.4
2E1	Clomethiazole	12
3A4/5	Ketoconazole	0.0037−0.18

Further detailed kinetic analysis of CYP activity can also be done with purified recombinant preparations of various CYPs.

Up to this point, the discussion has centered on what the liver can do to the drug; it is equally important to know what the drug can do to the liver. As mentioned previously, the liver is the first line of defense against foreign chemicals. As such, it receives high concentrations of exogenous xenobiotics which could compromise normal hepatic function. If this occurs due to drug treatment, serious health problems could result. Moreover, frequently patients are on multiple regimens of more than one drug and those treatments will have been titrated to the patient for safe therapy. Thus the patient can be considered a steady-state system where the rate of entry and exit of these drugs have been optimized to achieve a steady-state therapeutic level of drug. Therefore, anything that perturbs that steady-state may cause harm, either by allowing the minimum concentration to fall below therapeutic levels or by elevating concentrations into a toxic range. If this is caused by the introduction of another drug, this is referred to as a drug–drug interaction. It has been estimated that drug–drug interactions leading to toxicities are among the most prevalent causes of death in the United States, resulting in over 100,000 deaths a year. Determining the proclivity of a new drug entity to cause such interactions is a major function of the development process. One of the most common causes of drug–drug interaction is common activity at the hepatic system.

There are two ways in which one drug (considered here as the perpetrator) can affect the hepatic metabolism of another drug (considered as the victim). One is by functioning as a substrate for the same CYP as the victim (thereby reducing the metabolism of the victim). For example the antidiabetic drug metformin increases exposure to the antifungal itraconzole by 167% as both drugs are substrates for CYP3A1/2.[6] Another way in which hepatic drug–drug interactions can occur is if the perpetrator functions as a CYP inhibitor. This type of effect is separated into two types of activity. The first is a simple reversible inhibition which may or may not be debilitating; the point is that it subsides when the drug is removed by clearance and the enzyme activity returns. A second, and more serious, type of inhibition is termed "mechanism-based" (also referred to as "time-dependent"–see Fig. 6.9). This is an essentially irreversible inhibition of the enzyme characterized by an extremely long onset of effect and no recovery upon removal of the perpetrator. Thus, the CYP is essentially poisoned and normal CYP activity can only be regained with new synthesis of enzyme. An example of such interactions is the effect of psoralens from grapefruit juice (see Box 7.7). The five major CYPs (CYP1A2, 2C9, 2C19, 2D6 and 3A4) are targeted for testing for drug–drug interactions and when this activity is observed, it must be eliminated from the candidate molecule through chemical modification. Just as with co-substrate mechanisms, blockade of CYP activity can lead to serious drug–drug interactions. For instance, potentially fatal levels of the antihistamine terfenadine can be produced by inadvertent inhibition of CYP3A4. This is a particularly serious effect leading to fatal cardiac arrhythmias from a condition known as *Torsades des pointes*; this activity caused the recall of Terfenadine from the market.

As noted previously, the liver is a reactive organ which can elevate its function in response to stress. This can also occur in response to drugs and many are known to actively induce CYP enzyme synthesis and activity; this effect is termed "enzyme induction." Enzyme synthesis is initiated within 24 hours of exposure and increases over 3–5 days. The effect decreases over 1–3 weeks after the inducing agent is discontinued. Induction can occur through increased transcription of CYP genes through

BOX 7.7

THE UNEXPECTED EFFECTS OF GRAPEFRUIT JUICE IN CLINICAL TRIALS

Grapefruit juice was often used as a vehicle for drugs and placebos in double-blind clinical trials, since the strong bitter taste masked the taste of drugs. This preserved the double-blind nature of the trial. However, grapefruit juice contains psoralens which produce "suicide inhibition" of CYP3A4 (a reactive intermediate forms a covalent bond to irreversibly inactivate the enzyme). This causes large increases in blood levels of drugs that are metabolized by CYP3A4, notably lovastatin (see below — data from [12]). Untoward reactions from this effect have been noted for midazolam, triazolam and buspirone (impaired CNS function) and felodipine (hypotension).

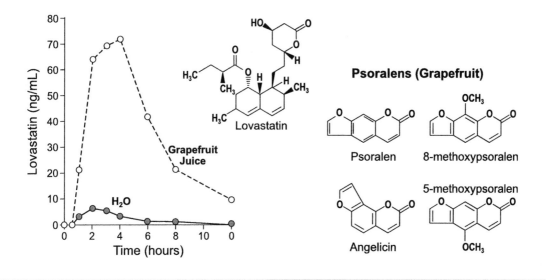

receptor-dependent mechanisms (PXR receptors) or stabilization of mRNA. Enzyme induction can seriously affect drug therapy. For instance, the already low oral bioavailability of the antihypertensive felodipine (15%) is reduced to near zero levels when administered with liver enzyme inducing anticonvulsants. However, as a general pharmacokinetic problem, it is (like plasma protein binding) not clear how it should be dealt with in early development. This is because it usually occurs at high doses (although some PXR effects can be seen at low doses) and it is extremely species-dependent. This latter fact makes it difficult to use animal models to predict how important the effect will be in humans. Enzyme induction can be determined *in vitro* through exposure of hepatocytes in cell culture over a prolonged period, homogenization of the cells to produce microsomes and observing any possible increase in enzyme activity or mRNA.

It can be seen how *in vitro* hepatic assays can be used to estimate drug metabolism, drug–drug interactions and liver enzyme induction. Figure 7.15 shows a decision tree illustrating a logical pathway for the testing of

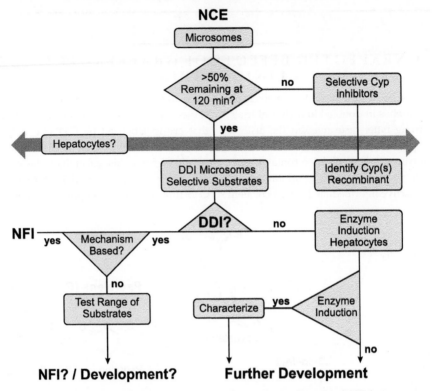

FIGURE 7.15　Decision tree for the study of hepatic effects of new chemical entities (NCEs). An assessment of stability in microsomes indicates whether the compound is a substrate for CYPs; if this is the case, then the CYPs can be identified through selective inhibitors or studied with recombinant enzymes. Irrespective of the outcome of this first step, the NCE must be assessed for possible proclivity to cause drug–drug interactions (DDI). If CYP is observed, then it must be determined whether it is mechanism-based. If so, development is halted. If not, it may still be unclear if the drug–drug interaction should preclude further development. If no drug–drug interactions are observed, the compound must still be tested for enzyme induction.

new molecules to assess their interaction with the hepatic system. In general it is important to test new chemical entities *in vitro*, because this may allow detection of reactive intermediates, identification of major metabolite(s) (which could then be synthesized and tested for activity) and the collection of data could aid in the selection of species for toxicological testing (which, in turn, would cover all human metabolites formed). In addition, metabolites formed only in humans could be detected; if this occurs, this identifies molecules that would be more costly to develop since there

would be no animal species to test for relevant toxicology.

ORAL BIOAVAILABILITY

One of the most common routes of drug administration is via the oral route and oral bioavailablility poses special problems in pharmacokinetics. This is because the drug must be absorbed through the GI tract wall where it immediately gets shunted to the portal vein and into the liver. Thus, the drug encounters two pharmacokinetically challenging processes; absorption and metabolism; this challenge is given the name "first pass effect" (Fig. 7.16). The total fraction of drug entering the central compartment via the oral route (denoted "F") is a product of the fraction absorbed (f_a) and the fraction that escapes the passage through the liver (f_h). Thus, $F = f_a \times f_h$, meaning that if 50% of the drug is absorbed and 50% emerges from the liver then the total oral bioavailability will be 25%. Data from two *in vitro* pharmacokinetic assays can be of use in predicting oral bioavailability; specifically permeation assays and measures of stability in liver microsomes, S9 and/ or hepatocytes. Clearly, a molecule that permeates cell layers quickly ($P_{app} > 10^{-5}\,\mathrm{cm\,s^{-1}}$) and is stable in hepatic *in vitro* cell preparations (> 50% parent compound remaining at 120 min) will have the highest probability of being an orally bioavailable drug. Figure 7.16

shows how plotting these values yield a grid where the top right quadrant isolates potentially bioavailable drugs during the compound sorting process in drug development. Since the drug is passing through the gastrointestinal tract there are other effects that enter into the calculation of *in vivo* bioavailability; these will be discussed further in Chapter 8. For instance, solubility in water is critical (see discussion of MAD and equation 7.1). Experimentally, a value for F of 0.2 is adequate while 0.5 is very good. However, there are exceptions to this rule. For example the F value for Etidronate, a bisphosphonate for stabilization of bone matrix in osteoporosis, is 0.03; in spite of this very low oral bioavailability, this is a viable drug treatment. In general, if values of $F > 0.2$ are not attained there are strategies to improve permeation, solubility or stability; these are outlined in Table 7.3.

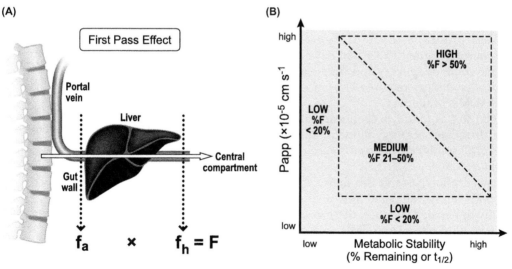

FIGURE 7.16 Oral bioavailability and the first pass effect. (A) Drugs given by the oral route are absorbed through the gastrointestinal wall and immediately enter the portal vein. This takes the drug to the liver before it can access the central compartment. (B) *In vitro* assays relevant to this process are permeation (passive diffusion in PAMPA or biological permeation in CaCo-2 cells; ordinate axis) or metabolic stability (microsomes, S9, hepatocytes) through readings such as percentage of parent compound remaining after 60 minutes incubation (abscissae). Compounds with corresponding values in the upper right corner would be expected to have favorable oral bioavailability. Those in the lower right or upper left would be expected to have poor oral bioavailability.

TABLE 7.3   Strategies for Improving Oral Bioavailability

Problem	Assay	Solution?
• Low solubility or slow dissolution	• Kinetic solubility assay	Reduce lipophilicity/make salts
• Low GI tract stability	• Stability in acidic buffer	Replace unstable groups
• Low metabolic stability	• Microsomes • Hepatocytes	Reduce lipophilicity/block metabolic sites
• Poor absorption due to low passive diffusion	• PAMPA • CaCo-2	Remove charges/hydrogen bond donors and acceptors/increase lipophilicity
• Poor absorption due to active efflux (P-gp)	• CaCo-2 (B→A)/(A→B)	Overwhelm by improving passive diffusion/remove or alter hydrogen bond acceptors/lower molecular weight
• Extensive biliary excretion	• *In vivo* assays	Reduce molecular weight/remove anionic charge/block conjugation

SUMMARY

- The structure–activity relationships for drug primary activity, pharmacokinetic properties (ADME) and safety profile can be different from each other.
- Modern drug discovery begins considering ADME at the very beginning of the discovery process.
- A discovery program likely will have limits set as to route of delivery and frequency of dosing; this defines required clearance and other ADME properties.
- The first step is to utilize chemical scaffolds with "drug-like" activity; defined limits of LogP, H_2O solubility, pK_a and molecular weight.
- Drug absorption (passive diffusion, transport) can be estimated *in vitro* as can stability to hepatic enzymes; these assays can be used to optimize ADME profiles.
- In addition there are *in vitro* assays available to determine whether a molecule inhibits hepatic enzyme function (this can be predictive of drug–drug interactions) or produces induction of live enzymes.
- Oral bioavailability results from a dual process of absorption followed by metabolism (first pass effect).

QUESTIONS

7.1 An active scaffold was found to be very insoluble in water. The team decided that this would "not be a problem" as an emulsion could be given that would be absorbed. Why are they wrong?

7.2 A drug discovery team was asked if they needed ADME support early in their program and they declined stating "we can build in the ADME properties after we get the lead." Why are they wrong?

7.3 What are some *in vitro* assays available to estimate the stability of molecule to hepatic degradation?

7.4 Why are discovery teams so worried about drug–drug interactions?

7.5 A drug candidate was tested in rats via the oral route after it was found to have a huge rate of permeation (38 cm s^{-1}) in the CaCo-2 *in vitro* permeation assay. The drug was not even detectable in rats indicating no bioavailability; what could be happening?

7.6 An investigational drug is found to cause the effect of another drug being used to treat the patient to lose its effect. What is one mechanism that can cause this effect?

References

[1] U. Velaparthi, P. Liu, B. Balasubramanian, J. Carboni, R. Attar, M. Gottardis, A. Li, A. Greer, M. Zoeckler, M.D. Wittman, D. Vyas, Imidazole moiety replacements in the 3-(1H-benzo[d]imidazol-2-yl)pyridin-2(1H)-one inhibitors of insulin-like growth factor receptor-1 (IGF-1R) to improve cytochrome P450 profile, Bioorg. Med. Chem. Lett. 17 (2007) 3072–3076.

[2] J.R. Proudfoot, Drugs, leads, and drug-likeness: An analysis of some recently launched drugs, Bioorg. Med. Chem. Lett. 12 (2002) 1647–1650.

[3] C.A. Lipinski, Drug-like properties and the causes of poor solubility and poor permeability, J. Pharm. Tox. Meth. 44 (2000) 235–249.

[4] C.A. Lipinski, F. Lombardo, B.W. Dominy, P.J. Feenery, Experimental and computational approaches to estimate solubility and permeability in drug discovery and development settings, Adv. Drug Delivery Rev. 23 (1997) 3–25.

[5] J.A. Galloway, R.E. McMahon, H.W. Culp, F.J. Marshall, E.C. Young, Metabolism, blood levels and rate of excretion of acetohexamide in human subjects, Diabetes 16 (1967) 118–127.

[6] Y.H. Choi, U. Lee, B.K. Lee, M.G. Lee, Pharmacokinetic interaction between itraconazole and metformin in rats: Competitive inhibition of metabolism of each drug by each other via hepatic and intestinal CYP3A1/2, Br. J. Pharmacol. 161 (2010) 815–829.

[7] R.S. Al-awar, J.E. Ray, R.M. Schultz, S.L. Andis, J.H. Kennedy, R.E. Moore, J. Liang, T. Golakoti, G.V. Subbaraju, T.H. Corbett, A convergent approach to cryptophycin 52 analogues: Synthesis and biological evaluation of a novel series of fragment a epoxides and chlorohydrins, J. Med. Chem. 46 (2003) 2985–3007.

[8] I. Kola, J. Landis, Can the pharmaceutical industry reduce attrition rates? Nature Rev. Drug Disc. 3 (2004) 711–716.

[9] W. Curatolol, Physical chemical properties of oral drug candidates in the discovery and exploratory development settings, Pharm. Sci. Tech. Today 1 (1998) 387–393.

[10] R.W. Clark, R.B. Ruggeri, D. Cunningham, M.J. Bamberger, Description of the torcetrapib series of cholesteryl ester transfer protein inhibitors, including mechanism of action, J. Lipid Res. 47 (2006) 537–552.

[11] N.A. Kasim, M. Whitehouse, C. Ramachandran, M. Bermejo, H. Lennernäs, A.S. Hussain, H.E. Junginger, G.L. Amidon, Molecular properties of WHO essential drugs and provisional biopharmaceutical classification, Mol. Pharm. 1 (2004) 85–96.

[12] T. Kantola, K.T. Kivistö, P.J. Neuvonen, Grapefruit juice greatly increases serum concentrations of lovastatin and lovastatin acid, Clin. Pharmacol. Ther. 63 (1998) 397–402.

Pharmacokinetics II: Distribution and Multiple Dosing

OUTLINE

By the end of this chapter the student will be able to put *in vitro* pharmacokinetic data on absorption and metabolism into the context of the *in vivo* environnment. The student will also understand *in vivo* clearance and volume of distribution, and how these factors control all of pharmacokinetics. Finally, the student will be able to see how data from a limited number of *in vivo* experiments can be used to generally describe the pharmacokinetics of any drug. These data also can be used to predict pharmacokinetics in other species to further predict dosing in humans for clinical study.

DRUGS IN MOTION: *IN VIVO* PHARMACOKINETICS

As shown in the previous chapter (see Fig. 7.4), a drug is nearly in constant motion from the instant it is introduced into the body until the time it leaves. Thus, the therapeutic target essentially responds to a running stream of drug of varying concentration. Chapter 9 discusses how this is relevant to the therapeutic response *in vivo*; this present chapter relates to the factors controlling the characteristics of that motion, what drug properties affect it and how they can be measured and quantified.

NEW TERMINOLOGY

The following new terms will be introduced in this chapter:

- **Allometric scaling**: The process of using body weight to predict physiological parameters in different animal species.
- C_{max}: The maximal peak concentration of drug observed in the central compartment as a result of a given dosing regimen.
- C_{min}: The minimal concentration of drug observed in the central compartment during repeat dosing.
- **Enterohepatic circulation**: The secretion of substances from the liver into the bile duct; these substances then can be reabsorbed from the gastrointestinal tract back into the body.
- **Extraction ratio**: The amount of substance removed from a flow of drug into a removal organ (i.e., liver) expressed as a ratio of the quantity entering the organ.
- **MRSD**: Maximal recommended starting dose for a human clinical trial.
- **NOAEL**: No observed adverse effect level for a drug.
- **NOEL**: No observed effect level for a drug.
- **Non-linear pharmacokinetics**: The pharmacokinetics seen *in vivo* when the clearance capacity of the body begins to be exceeded by the drug levels in the central compartment.
- τ: The dosage interval, i.e., the period between dosing in repeat dosing studies.
- **Volume of distribution**: The virtual volume of water in which drug appears to be dissolved when concentrations are measured in the central compartment; it can be used to detect sequestration of drug in various parts of the body.

THE CENTRAL COMPARTMENT AND *IN VIVO* CLEARANCE

The process of permeation and absorption controls the rate of entry of a drug into the central compartment; once there, immediate factors begin the process of drug clearance from the body and/or other processes that make the drug inaccessible to the therapeutic target. One of those, namely plasma protein binding, has been discussed briefly in Chapter 7. This process sequesters drug away from metabolic and renal processes of removal; it will be seen later in this chapter that plasma protein binding keeps the drug in the central compartment and does not allow it to be sequestered into other tissues. This has the effect of reducing the volume of distribution of the drug (*vide infra*). While plasma protein binding reduces free drug concentration, generally it is not a problem that needs to be addressed through medicinal chemical alteration of the molecule (see Box 8.1). This is because dosing is usually adjusted to accommodate it and limitations in free drug concentration are somewhat offset by a reduction in clearance afforded by plasma protein binding. For example, the antimuscarinic antagonists Zamifenacin and Darifenacin are of comparable potency (between two- to four-fold differences in IC_{50}) but differ by a factor of 300 in their plasma protein binding (Darifenacin is 94% protein bound while Zamifenacin is 98.98% protein bound). In spite of this radical difference in plasma protein binding, the equieffective clinical doses of Zamifenacin and Darifenacin differ by only a factor of two. In addition, the physico-chemical changes needed to change plasma protein binding are usually extensive and probably would interfere with primary activity or other ADME properties. The one realm where plasma protein is important is when clinical dose is compared to observed

BOX 8.1

IS DRUG PLASMA PROTEIN BINDING REALLY A PROBLEM?

While plasma protein binding can cause dissimulations between observed dosage of effective drugs and the concentration in the biophase actually producing the effect, it is not considered a roadblock to the development of drug therapies. Below are shown 43 of the 100 most prescribed drugs in the USA; it can be seen that over half are >90% plasma protein bound and some are >99.99% protein bound. In spite of this, the dosage administered accounts for this effect and these are useful therapies.

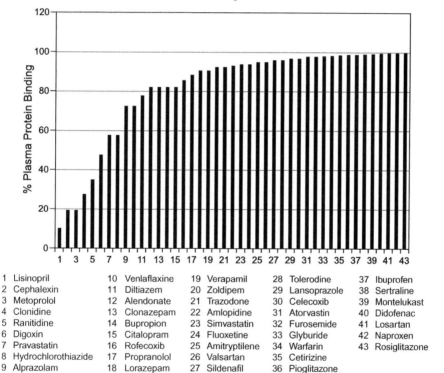

1 Lisinopril	10 Venlaflaxine	19 Verapamil	28 Tolerodine	37 Ibuprofen
2 Cephalexin	11 Diltiazem	20 Zoldipem	29 Lansoprazole	38 Sertraline
3 Metoprolol	12 Alendonate	21 Trazodone	30 Celecoxib	39 Montelukast
4 Clonidine	13 Clonazepam	22 Amlopidine	31 Atorvastin	40 Didofenac
5 Ranitidine	14 Bupropion	23 Simvastatin	32 Furosemide	41 Losartan
6 Digoxin	15 Citalopram	24 Fluoxetine	33 Glyburide	42 Naproxen
7 Pravastatin	16 Rofecoxib	25 Amitryptilene	34 Warfarin	43 Rosiglitazone
8 Hydrochlorothiazide	17 Propranolol	26 Valsartan	35 Cetirizine	
9 Alprazolam	18 Lorazepam	27 Sildenafil	36 Pioglitazone	

response and the true potency (and safety margin) of drugs needs to be calculated. This will be considered further in the next chapter (Chapter 9) on the measurement of pharmacologic effect *in vivo*.

Another way in which the central compartment drug concentration can change is through metabolic destruction; this is particularly true of esters as there are plasma esterases present to degrade esters to carboxylic acids. For example, the anticholinergic mydriatic drug eucatropine is destroyed in human plasma within 35 minutes. Similarly, the local anaesthetic procaine is destroyed in only a few minutes.

In addition to these factors, there are three forces moving drugs out of the central compartment (see Fig. 7.4), these are: (1) distribution to other compartments in the body; (2) renal excretion and (3) hepatic metabolism. Of these, hepatic metabolism is usually the most important and this will be considered first.

The body is a non-equilibrium system where drugs enter at a certain rate and are removed at a certain rate; the removal of a drug from the body is referred to as drug clearance. Drugs can be cleared through numerous organs in the body (i.e., liver, kidney, brain, lungs, sweat glands, etc.) and these are all treated as processes connected in parallel, except for the lungs which are considered a series process. Drugs introduced via the oral route undergo first pass metabolism (absorption from the gastrointestinal tract and then immediate shunting via the portal vein into the liver) while drugs introduced into the central compartment by other routes of administration are mainly cleared by the hepatic or renal system. The central compartment is cleansed of drug by cyclic filtering through either the liver or kidney (or both) until the drug is eliminated (see Fig. 8.1). In practical terms for non-polar drugs, the main organ of clearance is the liver. The efficiency of the liver as a removal organ can be quantified by an extraction ratio (E_H) given by:

$$\text{Extraction ratio} = E_H = 1 - \frac{[\text{concentration out}]}{[\text{concentration in}]}$$
$$(8.1)$$

Thus, if a concentration of 1 mg/L enters the liver and 0.3 mg/L emerges, this would be an extraction ratio of $1 - (0.3/1) = 0.7$, i.e., 70% of all drug that enters the liver is metabolized. Clearance is the rate of complete cleansing of a given volume of body water per unit time. Thus, if the liver receives 20 mL/min • kg of blood (this is the Q_H of the liver blood flow for a healthy adult) and a removal process extracts 70% of this, then the hepatic clearance (CL_H) is given by $Q_H \times E_H = 20$ mL/min kg $\times 0.7 = 14$ mL/min kg. For a 70 kg male this equals 980 mL/min. It is useful to denote levels of clearance in general terms as a fraction of liver blood flow. For a healthy male, liver blood flow is 1450 mL/min. Thus, a clearance value of 0 to 40% of liver blood flow is considered low (<580 mL/min), 40–70% medium (580 to

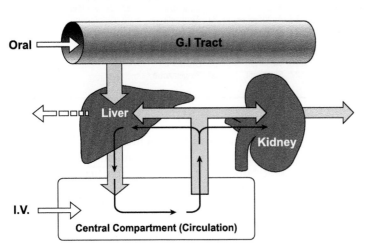

FIGURE 8.1 Clearance. Scheme depicting routes of elimination of drugs entering the body orally or directly from the central compartment. Oral drugs must pass through the liver before they enter the central compartment. The central compartment is then cleansed of the drug through repeated circulation(s) through the liver and kidneys until the drug is cleared from the body.

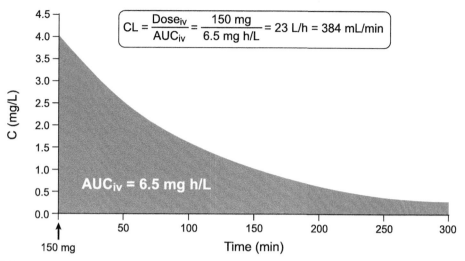

FIGURE 8.2 *In vivo* clearance. A single dose of drug given i.v. is allowed to completely clear from the body $(AUC_{iv} \rightarrow 0$ as $t \rightarrow \infty)$. The calculated area under the curve (AUC) for this drug is 6.5 mg hr L^{-1}. The dosage (150 mg) divided by this value yields the clearance which, in this case, is 384 mL min^{-1} (low).

1015 mL/min) and >70% (>1015 mL/min) high clearance.

Clearance is extremely important in pharmacokinetics as it determines the dose rate for clinical infusions to achieve therapeutic steady-state concentrations and it determines the dosing schedule for repeat administration in chronic treatment. It is the single most important determinant of whether a drug is a once a day, twice a day, etc., treatment. It can be measured *in vivo* by comparing the exposure to drug (expressed as the area under the concentration–time curve) and the dosage; it should be noted when *in vivo* clearance is measured in this way there is no restriction as to mechanism, i.e., it may be a mixture of removal mechanisms including hepatic and renal. Thus, Clearance$_{invivo}$ is given by CL = Dosage$_{iv}$/AUC$_{iv}$ (see Fig 8.2).

One additional mechanism of drug clearance related to hepatic function is secretion into the enterohepatic circulation. The liver secretes from 0.25 to 1 L of bile each day containing anions, cations and low molecular weight (<300) non-ionized molecules. The lower molecular weight compounds are reabsorbed before being excreted into the bile duct, but molecules of high molecular weight (approximately 500 or greater) can be secreted into the bile duct and continue on to be deposited into the gastrointestinal tract. The glucuronide conjugates of small polar structures can attain these sizes and glucuronides are known to take part in enterohepatic excretion. A practical aspect of this for clinical trials (and therapy) is the observation that some drugs that take part in this process (i.e., chloramphenicol; see Box 8.2) can demonstrate large secondary oral absorption curves after a meal as the bile is secreted into the GI tract in response to food.

RENAL EXCRETION

A main pathway for drug excretion from the body is through the kidney; this is the primary method of clearance for polar water-soluble chemicals. The kidney receives about 173 liters of water a day and returns approximately 171 liters back to the body. It filters water at a rate of

---

BOX 8.2

THE ENTEROHEPATIC CIRCULATION

The enterohepatic circulation forms a cycle whereby drugs are secreted into the bile duct (through transport processes such as P-gp, MDR2, MDR3, BSEP and MRP2) from the hepatic cells. They are shunted to the gastrointestinal tract when the gall bladder secretes bile (after a stimulus such as a meal) and from there they can be reabsorbed. This is known to occur with chloramphenicol and chloramphenicol-glucuronide. These effects must be considered in clinical trials where fasting conditions can affect absorption.

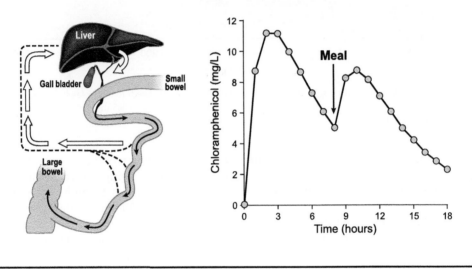

---

110 to 130 mL min^{-1} through a system of approximately one million nephrons (tubules) that have distinct properties (Fig. 8.3A shows one such tubule). Filtration begins at the glomerulus, an area of vasculature that has uniquely large pores that allow all but protein bound drug (> m.w. 30,000) to pass. The blood passes through the glomerulus at a rate of 1200 mL min^{-1} and 10% is filtered through as plasma water. The clearance by glomerular filtration is $CL_{GF} = f_u \times GFR$ where f_u refers to the free fraction of drug (non-protein bound) and GFR is the filtration rate (approximated at 120 mL min^{-1}). The filtrate then progresses to the proximal tubule which has secretory pumps capable of actively transporting drugs from the circulation into the tubule. There are two main secretory processes; one for negatively charged molecules (weak acids) and one for positively charged molecules (weak bases). This process is saturable and designated CL_S (see Fig. 8.3). Finally, in the loop of Henle, all but 1 or 2 mL of the 120 mL, filtered at the glomerulus, is reabsorbed. It is here that non-ionized membrane-soluble drugs are also reabsorbed according to a concentration gradient. This process is controlled by urine volume (high volume = low gradient = low reabsorption). Since only non-ionized drug is reabsorbed, pH and pK_a may become factors in how much drug is reabsorbed. In cases where urine pH is subject to change (i.e., pH is lowered in conditions of chronic

(A) **(B)**

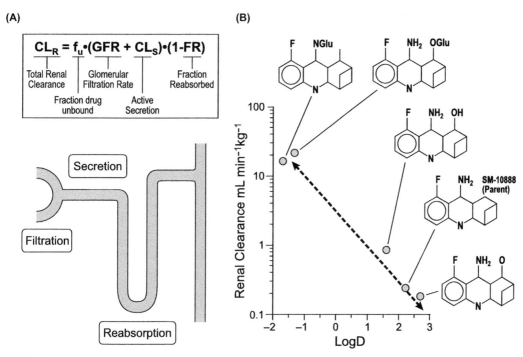

FIGURE 8.3 Renal clearance. Diagram on the left (A) shows a single renal tubule beginning at the glomerulus (where the process of plasma filtration occurs), to the collecting duct (which deposits urine into the bladder). Free drug is filtered at the glomerulus and it can also be actively secreted into the proximal tubule. As water passes down into the loop of Henle and distal tubule, it is reabsorbed. The graph on the right (B) shows the renal clearance of a parent drug (SM-10888), an acetylcholinesterase inhibitor, and its increasingly polar hepatic metabolites. It can be seen that as the LogD value for the metabolites decreases, the renal clearance correspondingly increases (data from [4]).

obstructive pulmonary disease, diabetic ketoacidosis, etc.), renal clearance may change for some drugs with disease state.

Considering all of the processes in the renal tubule, the total renal renal clearance is given by:

$$CLR = f_u(GFR + CLS) \times (1 - FR) \quad (8.2)$$

where: f_u is the fraction of non-protein bound drug; GFR is the glomerular filtration rate; CL_S is the amount of drug secreted into the tubule and FR is the fraction reabsorbed in the distal tubule and loop of Henle. Thus, if renal clearance is greater than GFR, the drug is secreted into tubules; if it is less than GFR, the drug is reabsorbed or highly protein bound. If renal clearance is equal to GFR then it is either freely filtered or the amounts secreted and reabsorbed

approach equality. In general, highly ionized drugs are filtered or secreted without being reabsorbed, causing them to appear rapidly in the urine. For example, p-aminohippuric acid is cleared in one passage through the kidneys (i.e., clearance is equal to the entire renal blood flow). Non-polar drugs are not as highly cleared by the renal system as they are reabsorbed. However, due to the fact that this process can be dependent on urine pH, this can be variable.

Renal clearance can be measured by:

$$CLR \ (mL/min) = \frac{Conc_U \ (mg/mL) \times U \ (mL/min)}{Conc_{plasma} \ (mg/mL)}$$

$$(8.3)$$

where $Conc_U$ and $Conc_{plasma}$ refer to the concentration of drug in the urine and plasma respectively and U refers to the rate of urine flow.

DRUG DISTRIBUTION

Referring to Fig. 7.4, it can be seen that another major process that a molecule undergoes, when introduced into the body, is redistribution. The body is comprised of numerous compartments, and drugs, owing to their particular physico-chemical properties, may sequester in some of these but not others. Knowledge of where drugs go in the body can be useful to determine the therapeutic potential of drugs; a tool to make these estimates is the volume of distribution (V_d). The volume of distribution of a drug is a virtual quantity of water into which a given drug would appear to be dissolved when the concentration is measured from the central compartment. Because the body is like a container with a hole in it, drug concentration changes with time. Therefore, to gauge the volume of distribution, the concentration at the instant the drug enters the body is required. This can be measured by estimating the clearance of a single intravenous dose of molecule. Figure 8.4A shows the decay in concentration with time of an intravenous dose of 20 mg of an experimental drug. This exponential decay curve can be linearized by plotting the natural logarithm of the

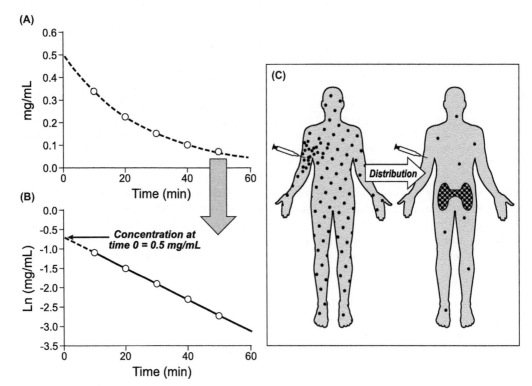

FIGURE 8.4 Volume of distribution. (A) A single dose of drug is given intravenously and the concentration with time is followed; an exponential decay is observed. (B) The ordinate drug levels are converted to natural log values to yield a straight line for the fall in concentration with time. This allows extrapolation to the theoretical concentration at time zero. This can be used to calculate the volume of distribution. (C) If a compound sequesters in a restricted compartment then the concentrations of drug will be low in the central compartment. This will yield a high volume of distribution.

concentration with time, as shown in Fig. 8.4B, allowing the extrapolation of the decay curve to time zero. This is the theoretical concentration of drug in the central compartment the instant the drug is injected. From this concentration value and knowledge of the amount of drug injected, the apparent volume of distribution of the drug can be calculated. In this case it is 20 mg ÷ 0.5 mg/mL = 40 L. This is approximately the amount of water in a 70 kg male, suggesting that the drug is evenly distributed in the body water. This procedure can be used to detect drug sequestration. For example, when 300 mg of the antimalarial drug chloroquine is given in a single intravenous dose, the concentration at time zero by extrapolation is 40 ng/mL (0.04 mg/L).[1] This leads to an estimation of V_d of 300 mg ÷ 0.04 mg/L = 7500 L, a volume approximately 180 times the volume of water in a human. This inordinately large V_d value indicates that chloroquine distributes to other tissues and is not present in the central compartment (see Fig. 8.4C). When drugs leave the central compartment and concentrate in other tissues (i.e., adipose tissue, muscle), the central compartment concentration will be exceedingly low and this, in turn, leads to an extremely high apparent volume of distribution. Therefore, high values for V_d are indicative of drug sequestration out of the central compartment. The factors that can cause drugs to be sequestered in special areas of the body (away from the central compartment) are entry into separated compartments such as the blood–brain barrier, mammary circulation, placenta, intracellular tissue binding, high lipid solubility and trapping due to pK_a/pH combinations. Binding of drugs to plasma proteins actually decreases the volume of distribution since it prevents free drug from diffusing elsewhere into the body.

There is a temporal aspect of the distribution of drugs within the body that leads to multi-compartment pharmacokinetics. The body is made up of many compartments of varying size, accessibility and blood flow, and access to these compartments varies with time. Upon injection, drugs rapidly distribute to highly perfused organs such as the liver, brain, kidney and lungs, over a time-scale of minutes. Over a period of hours thereafter, drugs then equilibrate according to their physicochemical properties throughout the body viscera (muscle, skin, fat). This leads to clearance curves that are more complex than those describing a single compartment. Figure 8.5 shows clearance from a three compartment system where the first two compartments are rapidly cleared to give a steep initial component to the curve; this profile represents redistribution of the drug within the body. The final phase of the curve represents true clearance where the drug leaves the body.

At this point it is useful to discuss the concept of half-time ($t_{1/2}$) with respect to whole body pharmacokinetics. The concentration of drug leaving a single compartment, as a function of time (denoted $[C]_t$), is given by:

$$[C]_t = [C]_0 \bullet e^{-k_{out}t} \qquad (8.4)$$

where: $[C]_0$ is the initial dosage given, t is time and k_{out} is a rate constant. This can be converted to a straight line through expressing the ratio $[C]_t/[C]_0$ as a natural logarithm ($Ln([C]_t/[C]_0) = -k_{out} \, t$). The time required for the concentration to fall to half its initial values ($[C]_t/[C]_0 = 0.5$; $Ln(0.5) = -0.693$) is denoted as the half-time ($t_{1/2} = -0.693/k_{out}$). Thus, since the $t_{1/2}$ directly relates to the rate constant for decay, it is a parameter that also characterizes the rate of decay. For a drug interacting with multiple compartments, a summation of processes according to equation 8.4, each with their own k_{out}, can model the curve. Figure 8.5 shows a three compartment system where the first two $t_{1/2}$ values represent redistribution while the third ($t_{1/2-3}$) represents true clearance from the body. While redistribution is important therapeutically and can pose clinical problems (e.g., retention of drug in rapidly

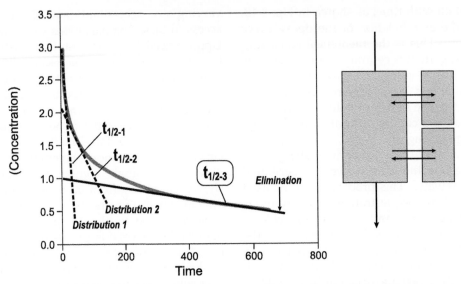

FIGURE 8.5 Drug clearance from a multi-compartment system. Shown is the central compartment drug concentration (ordinates) changing with time (abscissa) as the drug clears from the body. The drug redistributes from two low capacity but rapidly equilibrating compartments and then more slowly from a larger compartment. The rate of exit from each compartment can be approximated with a $t_{1/2}$ value; $t_{1.2-1}$ and $t_{1/2-2}$ quantify redistribution while true exit from the body is quantified by $t_{1/2-3}$.

distributed organs such as the brain for diazepam in *status epilepticus*), the main concern for drug development is whole body clearance. This is because the $t_{1/2}$ for removal of drug from the body dictates the duration of effect and frequency of administration.

A drug is considered cleared from the body after $5 \times t_{1/2}$ periods (>97% of the drug has left the body at that point). Similarly, if a drug is given repeatedly at intervals of every $t_{1/2}$, then it requires a period of $5 \times t_{1/2}$ to achieve steady-state concentration for therapy. For drugs which have an inordinately long $t_{1/2}$ (i.e., chloroquine), this dictates a long treatment period to achieve steady-state (see Box 8.3). The half-time of a drug in the body is an extremely useful characteristic number for a given drug and *in vivo* system; the application of this parameter to determine dosing regimens will be discussed in the next section.

If the therapeutic target resides in a compartment which has limited access (e.g.,

digoxin for cardiac cells) then the concentrations in the treatment compartment may be lower than those in the central compartment. They may also reach peak levels after peak levels in the central compartment have waned; this is shown in Fig. 8.6. Concentration is usually the driving force for flow into the restricted compartment, but *in vivo* drug levels are temporally transient, i.e., for i.v. dosing, concentrations begin high and diminish, while for oral dosing concentrations reach a peak within a given time and then also diminish. Therefore, the kinetics of central compartment concentration can be important to the restricted compartment, i.e., not only is the peak level important, but also how long the concentration remains high; Fig. 8.7 illustrates this effect. Panels 8.7A and B show a defined central compartment peak concentration with a resulting 10% peak concentration in a restricted compartment. Panel 8.7C shows the same drug in a system with a reduced rate of clearance;

BOX 8.3

LONG $t_{1/2}$ MEANS LONG PRETREATMENT TO STEADY-STATE

Just as 5 half-times represents the time it takes to nearly completely clear a drug (97%), it takes approximately 5 half-times to achieve a steady-state concentration of drug with repeated dosing if given every $t_{1/2}$. For drugs with very long half-times, this means that treatment may need to be prolonged to achieve a constant level of drug. Below is shown repeated dosing with a drug with an approximate $t_{1/2}$ of 40 hours (e.g.,

digoxin; gray tracing) and one with a $t_{1/2}$ of 200 hours (e.g., chloroquine; black tracing). Although these dosage intervals are not at $t_{1/2}$, the effect is similar, i.e., it takes considerably longer to achieve a steady-state with chloroquine than it does with digoxin. Chloroquine is an antimalarial and the long pretreatment requirement compels beginning of treatment 5 weeks before travel into a malaria-risk zone.

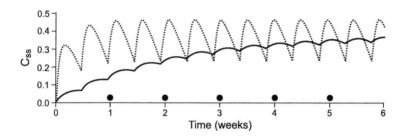

the dose has been reduced to mimic the peak concentration in Panel 8.7A. Note how this reduced clearance leads to a greater drug concentration in the restricted compartment (29%; see Fig 8.7D) in spite of the fact that the dosage has been reduced. This is because the concentration in the central compartment remains elevated for a longer time, allowing the slower diffusion into the restricted compartment to transfer more drug. This suggests that low clearance values for investigational drugs are optimal for transfer of drug into restricted compartments.

Drug distribution can be quantified with imaging. Using this technique, low energy molecules directly labeled with ^{11}C, ^{12}C, ^{18}F or ^{19}F are injected *in vivo* and imaged with positron emission tomography (PET). The

radionuclide emits positrons which are captured by a scanner; they are subsequently annihilated by electrons to yield gamma rays which are captured by a multiplier and used to construct an image. An example of how PET can be used for whole body pharmacokinetic studies is given in Box 8.4. An alternative method that does not require a radionuclide analog of the drug uses test molecules to displace a pre-labeled PET tracer already equilibrated in the organ of choice. This technique is not applicable to whole body pharmacokinetics but can be used to determine drug access to particular organs.

At this point it is worth putting the concepts of clearance and volume of distribution together to consider the *in vivo* pharmacokinetics of drugs. The aim of this endeavor is to

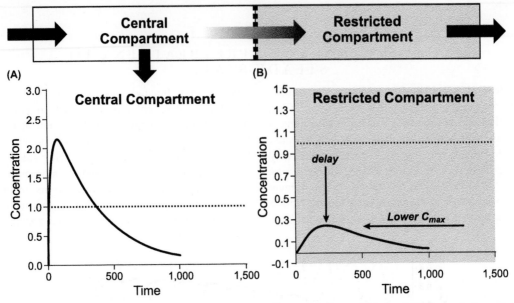

FIGURE 8.6 Drug diffusion into a restricted compartment. Top panel shows diffusion into the central compartment and subsequent diffusion from that into a restricted compartment. Panel (A) shows a hypothetical pattern of drug absorption and clearance in the central compartment. Panel (B) shows the resulting concentration of drug in the restricted compartment. Note how the peak is observed at a later time and is of lower magnitude than that in the central compartment.

characterize the pharmacokinetic parameters of a new drug entity to assess how it will behave therapeutically. Thus, "how much drug should be given" and "how often" are the critical questions with regard to how pharmacokinetics will control C_{ss}, the steady-state concentration of drug in the biophase available for therapeutic application.

PHARMACOKINETICS IN VIVO

Up to this point, the processes of absorption, metabolism and excretion have been treated somewhat as if they operate in isolation but, of course, in the body, they are concurrent and, sometimes, interdependent processes. As pointed out in Chapter 7, the steady-state drug level *in vivo* is due to a delicate balance of drug entering and leaving the system; anything that changes that balance could also change the steady-state. A great deal of knowledge about how these processes come together for a given drug can be obtained from minimal *in vivo* study (see Fig. 8.8). For example, the time course of plasma concentration of a single intravenous dose of compound can yield:

- clearance;
- volume of distribution;
- $t_{1/2}$.

Similarly, from a single oral dose, the following data can be obtained:

- F;
- t_{max};

where t_{max} is the time to peak concentration (a possible indicator of restricted absorption). It will be seen how these parameters can be used to form an idea about the *in vivo* stability of a compound and what dosing characteristics it will need to have in the therapeutic setting. In

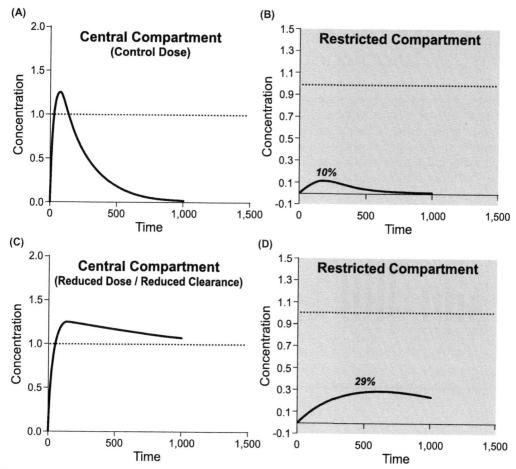

FIGURE 8.7   Diffusion into a restricted compartment as described in Fig. 8.6. Panels (A) and (B) describe a system resulting in a given set of values for absorption and clearance. Panels (C) and (D) show the same system with a reduction in clearance. The dose of the drug has been reduced to match the peak level in Panel (A). More of the central compartment concentration is able to enter the restricted compartment due to the fact that the reduced clearance allows the concentration to remain high for a longer period of time.

general, *in vivo* pharmacokinetic experiments can permit the study of metabolites, measurement of excretion (notably renal excertion) and can provide estimates of species-dependent plasma protein binding. In addition, the *in vivo* setting presents opportunities for observing drug–drug interactions not easily detected and studied *in vitro*. Finally, *in vivo* conditions may yield estimates of clearance and other pharmacokinetic parameters that are unique to a given

species or study condition; these must be identified and noted as exceptions when scaling is used to estimate pharmacokinetic parameters for humans.

Oral Bioavailability

Oral bioavailability (F) is directly measured as the ratio of AUC obtained by the oral route divided by the AUC produced by the same

BOX 8.4

VISUALIZING PHARMACOKINETIC COMPARTMENTS WITH IMAGING

Images of low energy analogs of molecules can directly indicate where molecules go in the body and the concentrations they attain in these compartments. Below are shown levels of the triazole antifungal Fluconazole (as a radioactive analog ^{18}F-Fluconazole) measured by quantita-tive positron emission tomography (PET) imaging. This technique allows quantitation of drug levels in different organs in the body and also shows real time drug level as it is cleared from the body (redrawn from [5]).

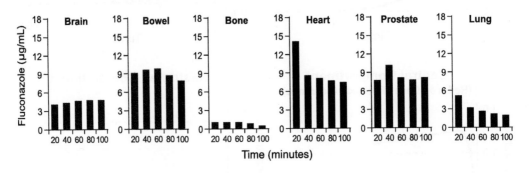

dosage given intravenously or, if the doses are different, then $F = (Dose_{iv} \times AUC_{po})/(Dose_{po} \times AUC_{iv})$. Thus, F values are the fraction of a dosage given via the oral route that makes its way into the central compartment (i.e., it is bioavailable). Experimentally, a value of F of 0.2 is adequate while 0.5 is very good. However, there are exceptions to this rule. As noted in Chapter 7, some bisphosphonates have extremely low F values yet, since they integrate nearly irreversibly into the bone matrix, eventually therapeutic levels accumulate. The AUC_{po} is proportional to the rate of drug absorption and the rate of clearance (usually hepatic); therefore any factor that alters these rates will alter the value of F for a drug. Table 8.1 shows some gastrointestinal tract effects that can subsequently affect oral bio-availability; in general, these stem from changes in the rate of absorption. These are uniquely *in vivo* effects that cannot be adequately predicted *in vitro*.

Drug–Drug Interactions

Drug–drug interactions are commonly encountered in the liver (see Chapter 7), but can also occur *in vivo* wherever drugs compete for saturable processes. Some of these interactions occur at the level of drug transport. For example, digoxin is a substrate for the efflux transporter P-gp, but dosage is adjusted to account for this. However, if a P-gp inhibitor is given *in vivo* (i.e., verapamil, quinidine,

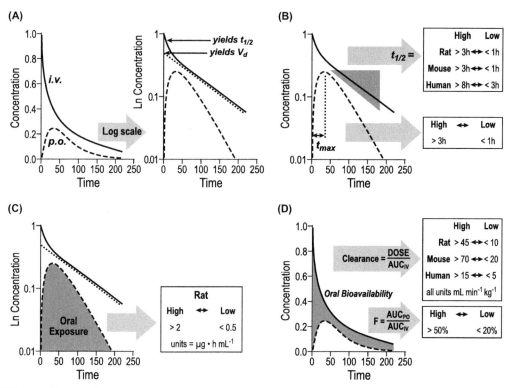

FIGURE 8.8 Pharmacokinetic parameters measured *in vivo*. (A) From a single intravenous dose the clearance, $t_{1/2}$ for elimination and volume of distribution can be calculated. With a single oral dosage, the time to peak maximum can also be measured. Panel (B) shows some characteristic values for rat, mouse and human. (C) A single oral dose also allows estimation of oral exposure. (D) A comparison of AUC_{oral} versus $AUC_{i.v.}$ allows a calculation of F. Shown are values for high and low F values in mouse, rat and human.

TABLE 8.1 GI Effects on Oral Bioavailability

	Increased	Decreased
Stomach emptying	i.e., hunger, exercise, metoclopramide	i.e. narcotics, antidepressants
	Increased absorption	Decreased absorption
Intestinal motility	i.e. gastroenteritis/decreased transit time	i.e. narcotics, anticholinergics, tricyclics
	Decreased absorption	Increased absorption
Chemical interaction	i.e. chelation of tetracyclines with metal ions	
	Decreased absorption	

TABLE 8.2 Some Drug–Drug Interactions Detected under *In Vivo* Conditions

Victim		Perpetrator	Mechanism	Outcome
Ketoconazole	+	Cimetidine	Altered gastric pH Altered GI transit	Reduced dissolution of ketoconazole; reduced absorption
Warfarin	+	Phenobarbitol	Induction of metabolism	Increased metabolism of warfarin → reduced anticoagulation
Theophylline	+	Cimetidine	Induction of metabolism Inhibition of metabolism	Cimetidine reduces clearance of theophylline leading to adverse effects
Digoxin	+	Hydralazine	Increased renal blood flow	Increased renal clearance of digoxin
Penicillin	+	Probenicid	Increased renal blood flow Increased tubular secretion	Prolonged half-life of penicillin allowing single dose therapy
Aspirin	+	Antacids	Increased renal blood flow Increased tubular secretion	Reduced tubular absorption of salicylate due to increased urine pH

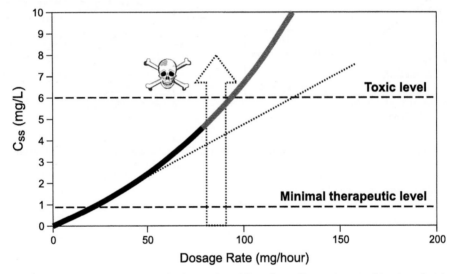

FIGURE 8.9 Non-linear pharmacokinetics. The linear dotted line shows linear pharmacokinetics whereby the capacity of the system to clear the drug is not saturated. Changes in dosage rate (abscissa) produce a correspondingly linear change in steady-state concentration of drug in the central compartment (C_{ss}). Under conditions of non-linear pharmacokinetics (where the capacity of the system to clear the drug is diminished with concentration), increased dosage rates cause an abnormally large increase in C_{ss}, as denoted by the curvature in the line.

cyclosporine-A), then digoxin toxicity can result as levels rise. Neurotoxicity to the anti-diarrheal loperamide is also observed when co-administered with quinidine. In general, when dealing with the complex physiology of the body, there are numerous ways in which one drug can interfere with the therapeutic action of another; some of these are given in Table 8.2.

Non-Linear Pharmacokinetics

The aim of pharmacokinetic studies is to derive predictions about central compartment

Linear Pharmacokinetics

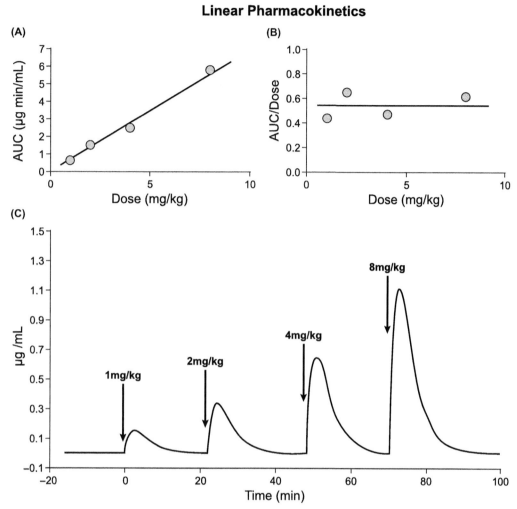

FIGURE 8.10 *In vivo* relationship between AUC and dose (Panel (A)) under conditions of linear pharmacokinetics. Panel (B) shows the horizontal relationship between AUC/dose ratios and dose. Panel (C) shows the actual AUC increases with dosage.

concentrations with a given dosage. A possible complication in this endeavor is the observation of "non-linear pharmacokinetics." While this may not lead to overt drug–drug interactions, this phenomenon can lead to capricious relationships between dose and drug blood levels. To discuss this further it is useful first to describe "linear" pharmacokinetics. This occurs when drug levels are well below the clearance capacity of the body. If clearance is approximated by a saturable process following Michaelis–Menten kinetics (i.e., hepatic clearance, renal transport) where the maximal velocity of the clearance is V_{max} and the sensitivity of the system to drug is K_M (this is the concentration of drug that half saturates the

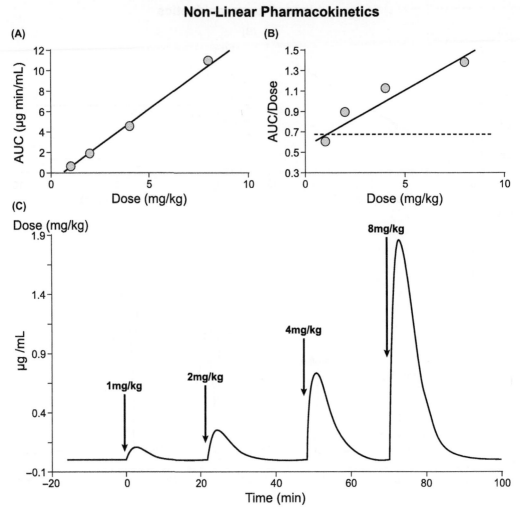

FIGURE 8.11   *In vivo* relationship between AUC and dose (Panel (A)) under conditions of non-linear pharmacokinetics. Note that the relationship between AUC and dose may still appear linear. Panel (B) shows that the relationship between AUC/dose ratios and dose is not horizontal. Panel (C) shows the actual AUC increases with dosage.

process), then the velocity of this process divided by the concentration of drug gives intrinsic clearance (CL_i):

$$CL_i = \frac{1}{[A]} \times \frac{[A]V_{max}}{([A] + K_M)} = \frac{V_{max}}{[A] + K_M} \quad (8.5)$$

It can be seen that when $[A] \ll K_M$ (when the concentration of drug is well below the

saturation point of the process), the $CL_i \approx V_{max}/K_M$. Since these are constant parameters of the system, the clearance is a constant, i.e., there is a constant rate of removal of drug (in vol/time units, e.g., mL/min) from the system. If the drug is given intravenously at a given dosage rate (e.g., DR infusion is µg/min), then the plasma steady-state

---

BOX 8.5
_____

NON-LINEAR PHARMACOKINETICS: WHERE MORE IS NOT NECESSARILY BETTER

There are a number of situations where *in vivo* pharmacokinetics are non-linear; many of these are encountered in the complicated process of oral dosing. Griseofulvin is an oral microcrystalline antifungal antibiotic used to treat fungal infections. It is nearly insoluble in water (12 mg/mL) and is dosed orally as a microsized or ultramicrosized powder. The limited solubility of griseofulvin in the gastrointestinal tract produces a unique profile with respect to dosing. Specifically, plasma levels with two capsules are actually higher than if four capsules are given (data drawn from [6]).

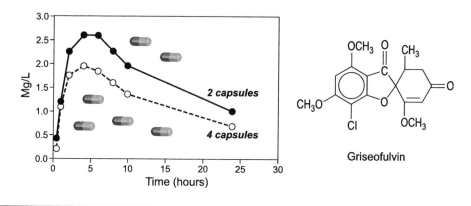

Griseofulvin

---

concentration is linearly related to the dosage rate (C_{ss} (μg/mL) = DR (μg/min) $\div$ Cl_i (μL/min)). This linear relationship can be used clinically to control therapeutic C_{ss} levels by adjustment of dosage rate (see Fig. 8.9). However, if the drug level rises to concentrations which begin to approach or exceed the capacity of the clearance system ([A] $\rightarrow$ K_M), the relationship between DR and CL_i becomes non-linear and follows equation 8.5 (Fig. 8.9). As this region of concentration is approached within the dosage rate, the normally linear curve becomes curvilinear and C_{ss} levels can become alarmingly high. This can become a problem in drug therapy and it also poses a problem for predictive pharmacokinetics.

Under conditions of linear pharmacokinetics, the exposure to a drug (as measured by the area under the plasma concentration–time curve) increases with drug dosage (see Fig. 8.10). However, the characteristic feature of AUC versus dosage with linear kinetics is that a plot of AUC/dosage versus dosage is a horizontal straight line (Fig. 8.10). Figure 8.11 shows conditions of non-linear pharmacokinetics. It can be seen that AUC may still increase with dosage and the line relating AUC versus dosage may even be straight, but this does not necessarily constitute linear pharmacokinetics. The important feature is to note that for this experiment, the plot of AUC/dosage versus dosage is not horizontal indicating that, as

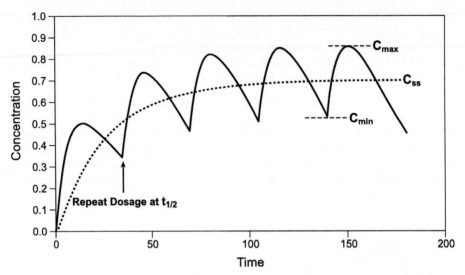

FIGURE 8.12   Repeat dosing at $t_{1/2}$ intervals leads to a steady-state concentration (C_{ss}) after approximately 5 $t_{1/2}$ periods. The actual temporal relationship between C_{ss} and time is characterized by a peak value (C_{max}) and a minimum value (C_{min}), also referred to as the trough.

dosage increases, clearance is diminishing (non-linear pharmacokinetics). It is essential to identify non-linear pharmacokinetics in the clinic as it can control how a drug is used therapeutically (e.g., control of plasma steady-state concentration with dosage rate, determination of time to steady-state, unresponsive recovery after cessation of dosing). In terms of drug development and the use of *in vivo* animal systems to predict pharmacokinetics in humans it is also important to detect such conditions, since non-linear kinetics can cause slow drug elimination (e.g., the $t_{1/2}$ for Phenytoin changes from 12 hours to 1 week) and an increased time to steady-state conditions. This can greatly decrease the predictive value of data from an *in vivo* system demonstrating non-linear pharmacokinetics.

There are a number of mechanisms *in vivo* that can lead to non-linear pharmacokinetics:

- **Decreased absorption**: Saturated gut wall transport (Riboflavin), saturated gut wall metabolism (Salicylamide).

- **Renal effects**: Active tubular secretion (Penicillin G), active tubular reabsorption (Ascorbic acid), alteration in urine pH (Salicylic acid), alteration in urine flow (Theophylline), nephrotoxicity (Gentamycin).
- **Effects on metabolism**: Capacity-limited metabolism (saturate the enzyme capability of metabolic system – Phenytoin), autoinduction (the compound induces its own metabolism by increasing CYP450 levels – Carbamazepine), co-substrate depletion (when co-substrate for conjugation is depleted leading to reduced elimination –Theophylline), product (metabolite) inhibition (Phenylbutazone).
- **Saturation of efflux transport**: e.g., P-gp saturation.

In addition to decreased absorption effects, non-linear pharmacokinetics can produce a decrease in bioavailable drug caused by problems with solubility (i.e., Griseofulvin; see

(A)

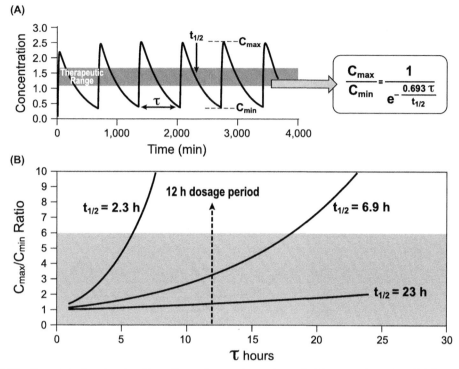

$$\frac{C_{max}}{C_{min}} = \frac{1}{e^{-\frac{0.693\,\tau}{t_{1/2}}}}$$

(B)

FIGURE 8.13 Repeat dosing showing C_{max}, C_{min} values and τ as the period between doses. Panel (A): Equation to the right shows the relationship between the ratio of C_{max}/C_{min}, $t_{1/2}$ and τ. Panel (B) shows C_{max}/C_{min} ratios as a function of τ for drugs of differing $t_{1/2}$. If the shaded area represents a maximum desired C_{max}/C_{min} ratio (higher ratios may indicate toxic concentrations or escape from minimal therapeutic concentrations), then it can be seen how a required dosage period of 12 hours limits the choice of molecule (based on $t_{1/2}$ values).

Box 8.5). This can be seen as an abrupt maximum in AUC with increasing dosage. For example, 100 mg/kg of the hepatoprotective agent YH439 produces an AUC of 32 mg min^{-1} mL^{-1} in rats; increasing the dosage to 500 mg/kg produces an AUC of only 37 mg min^{-1} mL^{-1}, indicating a limit to the solubility of this compound.[2]

The principal aim of pharmacokinetic studies is to estimate and model the ability of a new chemical entity to be adequately absorbed *in vivo* and to have the properties to allow it to remain in the bloodstream for a length of time suitable for therapeutic effect. This estimation can be made using observation of the effects of multiple dosing.

Figure 8.12 shows the effect of repeated oral dosing to achieve a level of C_{ss} (steady-state plasma concentration) adequate for therapy. It can be seen from this figure that if the drug is given at intervals of every $t_{1/2}$, then as discussed previously, a steady-state will be reached within five $t_{1/2}$ periods. This steady-state will still have variation in drug levels with time characterized by a C_{max} and a C_{min}. Clearly, the C_{max} must remain below predicted toxic levels while C_{min} (also called a "trough" concentration) must remain above minimally therapeutic levels. It is at this point that the importance of $t_{1/2}$ as a characteristic of a given *in vivo* system can be seen, as this parameter characterizes the ability of a drug

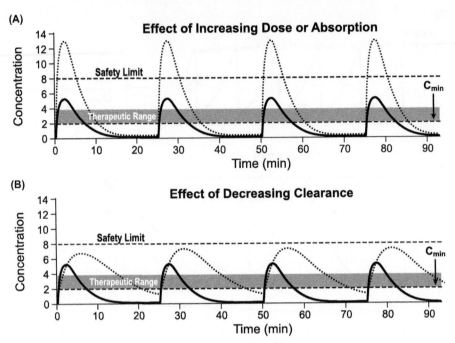

FIGURE 8.14 The effect of increasing dosage when the $t_{1/2}$ will not allow a convenient dosage period. Panel (A): It can be seen that little therapeutic coverage is gained from simply increasing the dosage under conditions of linear pharmacokinetics. Also, peak values may well extend beyond safety limits. (B) In contrast, a reduction in clearance can increase target coverage to a point where a substantially longer τ value can be attained.

to remain in the body for therapeutic effect. *In vivo* the $t_{1/2}$ is given by:

$$t_{1/2} = \frac{V_d}{\text{Clearance}} \qquad (8.6)$$

Thus, high clearance produces a low $t_{1/2}$ (rapid excretion from the body) while a low clearance yields a high $t_{1/2}$. Similarly, a high volume of distribution yields a high $t_{1/2}$ (large V_d values indicate sequestration of the drug in compartments with subsequently retarded efflux) and a low V_d a correspondingly low $t_{1/2}$.

The $t_{1/2}$ is a very important parameter as it links the original remit of a new drug discovery group and to what will need to be dealt with in the evaluation of experimental candidate molecules. Usually, the characteristics of a desired drug profile are known at the outset of a discovery program. For example, the chemical target may be an oral once-a-day treatment. The $t_{1/2}$ can be linked to dosage frequency and thus be used to assess candidate suitability. Defining a desired C_{min} for target coverage and also a C_{max} for safety, a ratio of C_{max}/C_{min} can be determined. This is related to the dosage rate (denoted as τ for the period between doses) by the $t_{1/2}$ with the following equation:

$$\frac{C_{max}}{C_{min}} = \frac{1}{e^{-\frac{0.693\tau}{t_{1/2}}}} \qquad (8.7)$$

This equation can be used to set useful guidelines for what the $t_{1/2}$ of an investigational compound needs to be for a given dosing regimen. Figure 8.13A gives a graphical representation of the parameters used for equation 8.7.

BOX 8.6

WHEN THERAPEUTIC EXTREMES MAY OVERCOME LIMITED PHARMACOKINETICS

Usually the half-time of a drug dictates the dosage frequency if the C_{max}/C_{min} ratio needs to be kept within a certain limit. High dosage may be used to increase C_{min}, but with this comes a correspondingly high C_{max} which could pose problems with safety. However, if the drug is inordinately safe, then it may be possible to give fairly large doses at intervals ($>>t_{1/2}$) that are more amenable to better patient compliance. This approach may give drug exposure periods of sufficient magnitude to be therapeutic. One such drug is Augmentin (amoxycillin/clavulanate combination) used for treatment of pediatric otitis.

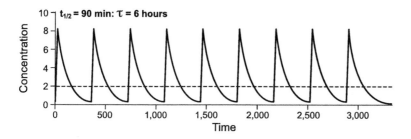

BOX 8.7

WHEN SLOWER IS BETTER

For drugs with marginal $t_{1/2}$ values, it may be difficult to reconcile adequate therapeutic coverage and a dosage regimen compatible with reasonable patient compliance. The left panel shows multiple dosing with a drug that is rapidly absorbed and cleared. A high dosage may provide target coverage but the fluctuation in concentration (C_{max}/C_{min} ratio) is unacceptably high. However, by reducing the rate of absorption (through coated tablets) and increasing the dosage, a better and less fluctuating steady-state concentration may be achieved

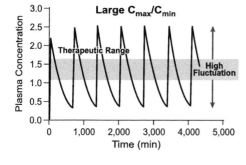 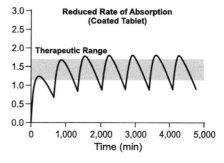

TABLE 8.3 Physiological Parameters of Various Animal Species

	Body weight	Blood flow liver (mL/min)	Kidneys (mL/min)	Urine (ml/day)	GFR[1] (mL/min)
Mouse	0.02 kg	1.8	1.3	1	0.28
Rat	0.25 kg	13.8	9.2	50	1.31
Rabbit	2.5 kg	177	80	150	7.8
Monkey	5 kg	218	138	375	10.4
Dog	10 kg	309	216	300	61.3
Human	70 kg	1450	1240	1400	125

	Total body water (mL)	Compartment Intracellular fluid (mL)	Volumes Extracellular fluid (mL)	Plasma volume (mL)
Mouse	14.5	–	–	1
Rat	167	92.8	74.2	7.8
Rabbit	1790	1165	625	110
Monkey	3465	2425	1040	224
Dog	6036	3276	2760	515
Human	42,000	23,800	18,200	3000

Figure 8.13B shows the C_{max}/C_{min} ratios for three molecules of varying $t_{1/2}$. In this example it can be seen that if a dosing period of 12 hours is required, then a compound with a short half-life ($t_{1/2} = 2.3$ h) would be completely inadequate.

Equation 8.7 can be useful for predicting dosage interval. For example, assume that an experimental HIV-1 entry inhibitor with a $t_{1/2}$ of 6 hours has a K_i for blocking HIV-1 entry of 100 nM. For protection against HIV-1 entry, it is proposed that a $10 \times K_i$ concentration would be needed in the target compartment at all times; for a molecule of molecular weight of 389, this would be a minimum concentration required for therapy (C_{min}) of 0.4 μg/mL. It is also known that a 10 mg dose gives a C_{max} value of 2.5 μg/mL, well below the toxic level of 10 μg/mL. Using

2.5 μg/mL as C_{max}, this sets C_{min}/C_{max} at 0.4/ 2.5 = 0.17 μg/mL. Rearranging equation 8.7:

$$\tau = \frac{-Ln\left[\dfrac{C_{min}}{C_{max}}\right] \bullet t_{1/2}}{0.693} \qquad (8.8)$$

which predicts a τ value of 15.3 hours. Thus, a 10 mg dose given every 12 hours should produce adequate target coverage for this investigational drug.

It is important to note that clearance is the major determinant of the dosing interval and that simply increasing the dosage of a highly cleared drug will not increase $t_{1/2}$ or the dosage interval τ. Figure 8.14A shows how increasing the dosage will increase C_{max} (up to possible toxic levels) but will only minimally increase the duration of effect. In contrast, Fig. 8.14B

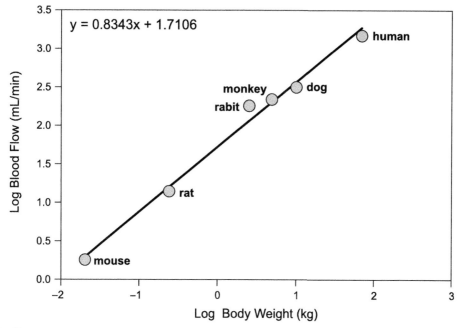

FIGURE 8.15 Allometric scaling. Graph shows a regression of Log liver blood flow on Log (body weight) according to the allometric scaling equation (equation 8.10). If hepatic metabolism is the primary method of clearance and is a constant percentage of liver blood flow in the range of species shown, then a graph of clearance in the animal species will be linear with the same slope, allowing prediction of clearance in humans.

shows how a decrease in clearance will subsequently enable increased τ and give better target coverage. There are cases where an increased dosage may be adequate if the periods of exposure are sufficient for target coverage and if the drug is very safe (see Box 8.6). Another strategy to achieve a suitable τ value to meet compliance is to use a formulation such as coated tablets to retard absorption to avoid high (and possibly toxic) C_{max} levels (see Box 8.7).

SCALING DATA TO PREDICT HUMAN PHARMACOKINETIC BEHAVIOR

In vitro and *in vivo* pharmacokinetic studies are usually done in a variety of animal species in an effort to characterize the ADME properties of a given molecule and also to predict the pharmacokinetics that will be observed in humans. An important tool in this endeavor is the process of allometric scaling. This is a method of predicting parameters in various species based on body weight. The basic equation for this is:

$$Y = a \cdot W^b \qquad (8.9)$$

where Y is the physiological parameter in question, a and b are fitting parameters and W is body weight. It is used in pharmacokinetics in the logarithmic form:

$$Log(Y) = Log(a) + b\,Log(W) \qquad (8.10)$$

The basis for this equation is the relationship between observed and calculated values

BOX 8.8

THE STATISTICAL GEOMETRY OF ALLOMETRIC SCALING

The main tool in allometric scaling is a linear regression of the equation (specific example for clearance):

$$Log(Clearance) = Log(A) + b \, Log(Body \, Weight)$$

Theoretically, any three animal species could define a straight line for scaling to values for humans. However, the error for the slope of a regression line is the rotation about the mean x and y values, and the further away the extrapolated value is from mean x and y, the greater the error in estimation. Therefore, it is usually imperative to have an animal species of larger body weight to define the regression line for an accurate estimate for humans (70 kg).

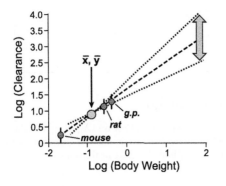 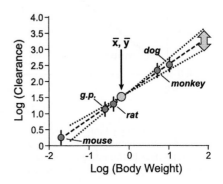

of physiological parameters and body weight; some of these are shown in Table 8.3. The liver blood flow of various species, as a function of body weight, is shown in Fig. 8.15; the straight line results from fitting the data to equation 8.10. The same can be done for most physiological parameters such as volume of distribution and renal clearance. From these relationships measurements taken in a range of species can be used to extrapolate the value for humans. If the molecule in question is cleared by the same mechanisms in all species, then scaling works well (although a larger body weight species is recommended for accurate scaling to humans; see Box 8.8). Allometric scaling can also be used to identify species that demonstrate idiosyncratic pharmacokinetics for a given compound. Figure 8.16 shows the scaling data for the antibiotic CS-023; it can be seen that the data for the monkey lies off the linear regression scaling line. Subsequent data showed that CS-023 is abnormally well reabsorbed in the kidney tubules of monkeys, thereby identifying the reason for the aberrant pharmacokinetics.[3]

Once sufficient studies have been undertaken to predict suitable pharmacokinetics in humans, the data is applied to estimate the starting dosage for human studies. There are numerous factors involved in this procedure affecting safety and predictability of effect; these include the NOEL (no observed effect level) and NOAEL (no observed adverse effect level) in animals. The NOAEL can be used to

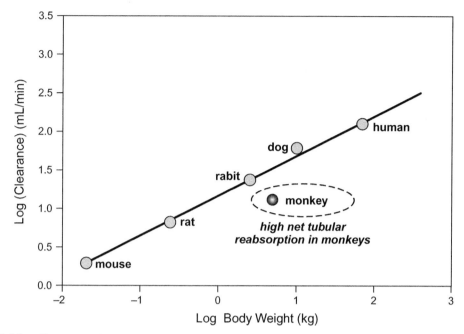

FIGURE 8.16 Allometric scaling regression for the antibiotic CS-023 clearance. While values for mouse, rat, rabbit, dog and human reside on the linear regression, values for monkey diverge. Subsequent study showed this species had an abnormally high net renal tubular reabsorption, causing an aberrant reduction of clearance in this species.[3]

predict the MRSD (Maximum Recommended Starting Dose) in humans by:

$$MRSD = NOAEL_{animal} \bullet \left[\frac{SA_{human}}{SA_{animal}} \right]$$
$$\bullet \left[\frac{1}{10} Safety\ Factor \right] \quad (8.11)$$

Where SA refers to body surface area given by:

$$Body\ Surface\ Area\ (m^2) = 1.85 \bullet \left(\frac{W}{70} \right)^{2/3} \quad (8.12)$$

In general, Chapters 7 and 8 have described the types of *in vitro* and *in vivo* experiments that can be done to characterize the ADME properties of new chemical entities. Figure 8.17 summarizes the steps that can be taken *in vivo*, first with single and then with multiple dose studies to determine *in vivo* pharmacokinetics. These data can then be used in allometric scaling experiments both to choose the appropriate species for toxicology and efficacy studies, and also to project how best to progress to testing in humans.

SUMMARY

- The kidney filters and excretes polar water-soluble compounds. Non-polar compounds are filtered but may be reabsorbed.
- The extent of distribution of a drug can be determined by measuring the volume of distribution.
- Reduction in whole body clearance can be useful to increase drug distribution into restricted body compartments.
- Observing the decay, with time, of drug levels from a single i.v. dose can yield estimates of clearance, volume of

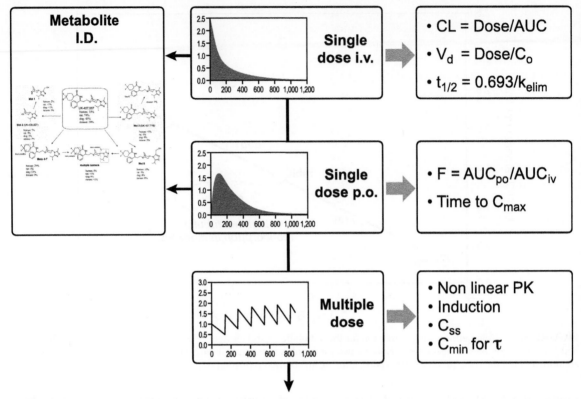

FIGURE 8.17 Summary of *in vivo* pharmacokinetics studies. Intravenous and oral doses can provide estimates of clearance, volume of distribution, $t_{1/2}$, t_{max} and F. Analysis of plasma samples in different species also allows identification of metabolites. Multiple dose studies allow detection of non-linear pharmacokinetics, possible induction effects, C_{ss} and estimation of τ values.

distribution and $t_{1/2}$. A single oral dose can yield values for oral absorption (F).

- While there are *in vitro* experiments that can yield data to characterize specific processes relevant to *in vivo* pharmacokinetics (i.e., absorption, metabolism), there are factors encountered *in vivo* that can modify *in vitro* predictions.
- For example, solubility and other absorption effects in the gastrointestinal tract can modify the impact of first pass metabolism. Similarly, renal effects are not accounted for *in vitro*.
- *In vivo* experiments can detect complex mechanisms of drug–drug interactions and non-linear pharmacokinetics.

- Non-linear pharmacokinetics should be identified both as a therapeutic challenge and also as a factor in evaluating animal data to predict pharmacokinetics in humans and other species.
- Multiple dosing is used *in vivo* to achieve a therapeutic steady-state level of drug adequate for therapy (C_{ss}). The $t_{1/2}$ for elimination is an important determinant of the frequency of dosing possible to achieve adequate C_{ss}.
- In general, the rate of drug clearance is the dominant factor in determining frequency of dosing needed to attain adequate C_{ss}.

- Allometric scaling is a procedure whereby the pharmacokinetic data obtained in a range of animal species can be used to predict the pharmacokinetics in humans.
- Allometric scaling can also be used to detect aberrant pharmacokinetics in any single species.

QUESTIONS

8.1 What is clearance?

8.2 A volume of distribution for a new drug was found to be 159 liters. How could this be if a human normally has about 40 liters of total body water?

8.3 Clinicians are able to control seizures in a patient through careful monitoring of an intravenous drip. As the dosage increases, suddenly the concentration of drug in the patient rises sharply to overdose levels; what could be happening?

8.4 A drug is given as a single i.v. injection and the concentration monitored. The initial $t_{1/2}$ is 5 minutes, suggesting a rapid elimination, but this changes to a $t_{1/2}$ of 2 hours. What happened?

8.5 A given investigational drug was extremely well absorbed via the oral route and had a $t_{1/2}$ of 9 hours (adequate for once-a-day dosing). Unfortunately, the safety margin for this compound was limited as toxic effects were seen at 2.5 times the C_{max} for the dose used. What is a strategy that could be employed to make this compound more reliable and therapeutically useful?

References

[1] L.L. Gustafsson, O. Walker, G. Alvain, B. Beermann, F. Estevez, L. Gleisner, et al., Disposition of chloroquine in man after single intravenous and oral doses, Br. Clin. Pharmacol. 15 (1983) 471–479.

[2] W.H. Yoon, J.K. Yoo, J.W. Lee, C.-K. Shim, M.G. Lee, Species differences in pharmacokinetics of a hepatoprotective agent, YH439 and its metabolites M4, M5, and M7 after intravenous and oral administration to rats, rabbits and dogs, Drug Metab. Disp. 26 (1998) 152–163.

[3] T. Shibayama, Y. Matsushita, A. Kurihara, T. Hirota, T. Ikeda, Prediction of pharmacokinetics of CS-023 (RO4908463), a novel parenteral carbapenemantibiotic, in humans using animal data, Xenobiotica 37 (2007) 91–102.

[4] D.A. Smith, B.C. Jones, D.K. Walker, Design of drugs involving the concepts and theories of drug metabolism and pharmacokinetics, Medicin. Res. Rev. 16 (1996) 243–266.

[5] A.J. Fischman, et al., The role of positron emission tomography in pharmacokinetic analysis, Drug Metab. Rev. 29 (1997) 923–956.

[6] M. Rowland, T. Tozer, Clinical Pharmacokinetics: Concepts and Applications, Lippincott, Williams & Wilkins, Baltimore, MD, 1995 (pp. 450–451).

9

In Vivo Pharmacology

By the end of this chapter the reader will understand the various pharmacokinetic and pharmacodynamic factors involved in the production of *in vivo* drug response, as well as some of the ways in which these can be quantified and predicted in simple *in vitro* experiments. Also readers will see that since the body is an open system (not in equilibrium) the kinetics of the interaction of drugs with targets becomes paramount and a major determinant of overall *in vivo* activity.

WHOLE BODY DRUG RESPONSE

The tremendous technological advances over the past 200 years in medicine and pharmacology overshadow the equally tremendous history of empirical drug discovery done *in vivo* over the past 5000 years. Considering ideas set forth in the Ebers papyrus (a very early source of ancient "prescriptions;" see Box 9.1), the modern period of *in vitro* testing

comprises only 4—5% of the time empirical medicine has been practiced; the other 95—96% of the effort has been drug discovery done *in vivo*. Within this period the trial and error testing of herbal remedies forms a rich history of early drug discovery (e.g. see Withering and the Discovery of Digitalis; Box 9.2). In addition to observing desired therapeutic activity, the clinical testing of new drugs has led to observation of "side-effects" some of which provided insights into therapies for different diseases (see Box 9.3). With this history as a backdrop, modern pharmacology and drug discovery combines the rigor of *in vitro* testing (where drug concentration is known) and pharmacokinetic modeling of drug response *in vivo*. All the previous chapters are aimed at methods and strategies to obtain a molecule that will be therapeutically useful *in vivo*. This chapter considers the two topics of pharmacodynamics (primary activity at the therapeutic target) and pharmacokinetics (delivery of a therapeutic dose *in vivo* to the target organ) and combines

BOX 9.1

THE EBERS PAPRYUS: PRESCRIPTIONS FROM ANTIQUITY

The Ebers papryus (so called because it was purchased in Luxor by Georg Ebers in 1873) is one of the oldest surviving medical records known. Thought to be written in approximately 1500 BC, it contains nearly 700 "prescriptions" (some dating from 3000 BC) for the treatment of maladies. Although many of these prescriptions are magical formulas and remedies, some hold kernels of pharmacological logic. For example,

for night blindness, the "liver of ox" was suggested. Since night blindness can be caused by a deficiency in Vitamin A, and since liver is an excellent source of Vitamin A, this prescription should produce a useful effect. A partial translation of the Ebers papryus by Carpenter and colleagues[8] gives an intriguing example of ancient *in vivo* pharmacology.

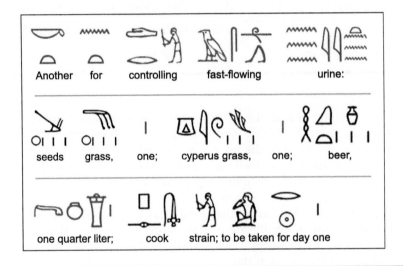

them to discuss the final *in vivo* activity of a drug. The third main element of discovery, namely safety pharmacology, will be discussed in the next chapter.

When a drug enters the body, it encounters a complex and dynamic system that has its own basal activity combined with reflex mechanisms designed to counter any perturbation. As seen in Fig. 9.1, a drug introduced orally must dissolve in the gastrointestinal tract, be absorbed through the lumen and pass

through the liver before it can enter the central compartment. Drugs introduced intravenously already gain access to the central compartment. From there, drugs can be destroyed by enzymatic degradation, bound by plasma proteins, distributed to other compartments of the body, be further destroyed by hepatic metabolism or be directly excreted by the renal (or other) system. During this process, quantities of drug in body compartments can interact with tissues to produce pharmacologic

BOX 9.2

WITHERING, DROPSY AND THE FOXGLOVE PLANT

While working at Birmingham General Hospital in 1779, the British physician William Withering noticed a woman with "cardiac dropsy" (fluid swelling from congestive heart failure) improve remarkably after ingesting a local herbal remedy. He learned about the remedy from an old woman herbalist and went on to determine that the active ingredient was digitalis. In the years following he systematically explored different preparations (gathered at various times of the year) to document 156 cases of the use of digitalis. In 1785 he published his famous paper "An Account of the Foxglove and Some of its Medical Uses." This treatise describes clinical trials and notes on the therapeutic effect of digitalis and its toxicity; it is a classic chronicle of *in vivo* drug discovery and development. This subject became a topic of dissention when a physician colleague of Withering, Erasmus Darwin, was called for a second opinion and published the paper "An Account of the Successful Use of Foxglove in Some Dropsies and in Pulmonary Consumption." This led them to become estranged and led to a bitter argument over what Withering considered academic plagiarism.

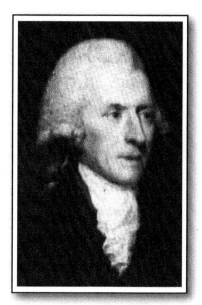

William Withering
(1741–1799)

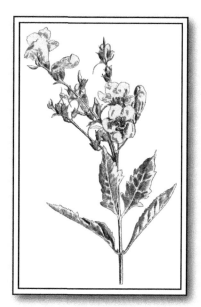

Foxglove
(Gerardia Quercifolia)

BOX 9.3

NEW DRUGS FROM SIDE-EFFECTS

One of the main problems in drug discovery is the need for drug-like properties and adequate safety in molecules to allow testing in humans for proof of concept. When a drug meets these criteria it can be an extremely useful tool for the exploration of other possible useful activities through the observation of secondary effects (so called "side-effects"). Thus, the observed diuresis with the antibacterial sulfanilamide led to the development of the diuretic furosemide. Similarly, the development of the antidiabetic tolbutamide arose from observations with the antibacterial carbutamide.

One of the most difficult areas of drug development is in diseases of the central nervous system. This is because of the subjectivity and complexity involved in the interpretation of CNS effects for diseases such as depression and psychosis. In the 1950s, efforts to develop antihistamines led to compounds that caused patients to be "disinterested in their surroundings." This CNS side-effect was recognized as possibly of value to patients who have constant unwanted sensory input in schizophrenia. This led to the development of chlorpromazine, the first drug for that disorder.

---

responses. Some of these may be beneficial (therapeutic response) and others may counter the therapeutic effect or produce other effects that may compromise normal cellular activity. These latter interactions can raise safety issues. In general, the observed response to a drug takes into consideration the pharmacokinetic factors that can affect the magnitude of the dose given, the integration of all the responses produced by the drug, the effect of body reflexes and finally, the interaction of the drug with the ongoing basal physiological activity of the system.

NEW TERMINOLOGY

- **Biomarkers**: An observed finding that can be associated with drug effect, disease or physiological state. These can be physiological readings, chemical or biochemical substances, or images.
- **ROC curves**: Receiver operated characteristic curves are used to evaluate procedures; in this case, the effectiveness of biomarkers as predictors of disease or drug effect.

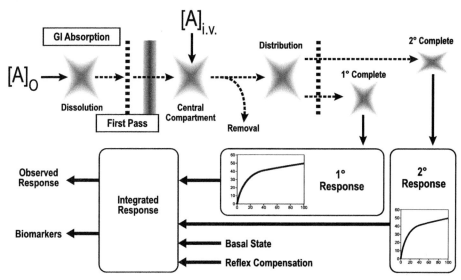

FIGURE 9.1 Schematic diagram of the route of travel of a drug given either intravenously (i.v.) or orally in an *in vivo* system. The production of observed effect is seen as a function of the primary therapeutic (desired) drug action modified by secondary effects, interaction with the basal physiological tone of the system and *in vivo* reflexes.

- **Target coverage**: A term that encompasses the degree to which and the length of time a biological target is associated with (bound to) a drug molecule.

THE "DOSE" IN DOSE–RESPONSE

Chapters 7 and 8 extensively consider the properties required of a molecule to reach the target organ in the body and be present there for a sufficient length of time to be therapeutically useful. There are examples of where pharmacokinetics can completely dominate how a drug works *in vivo* (see Box 9.4). This chapter will now relate the pharmacokinetically available dose with observed *in vivo* response. It should be recognized that drug levels are measured in the body from samples taken from the central compartment and these may be quite different from the drug levels in the compartment actually containing the biological target for therapy (see Fig. 9.2). There

are factors in the central and therapeutic compartment which can alter the concentration of drug producing an observed effect; two of these are plasma protein binding and restricted diffusion.

Plasma protein binding was discussed in Chapter 7 as a factor causing divergent values for dosages given *in vivo* and those that are actually free to produce a response. While not an extremely important factor in candidate selection of molecules, it can obscure whole body pharmacokinetics (see Box 9.5). It is also important when clinical dose is compared to observed response and the true potency (and safety margin) of drugs needs to be calculated. Plasma protein binding is a saturable process; therefore its importance may change with dosage level. Figure 9.3A shows the aberration of central compartment drug levels by plasma protein binding. It can be seen that as the drug level saturates the amount of protein available, the central compartment concentration approaches the dosage given. Depending on

BOX 9.4

THE ROUTE OF DRUG ADMINISTRATION CAN MEAN THE SAME DRUG CAN BECOME A DIFFERENT DRUG

The route of administration of a drug *in vivo* can be a means of increasing the delivery of the drug to a given organ to optimize the active concentration at the therapeutic target. It can also effectively reduce the side-effects to a drug *in vivo*. For example, β-adrenoceptor bronchodilators in asthma reach the constricted bronchioles at a maximal concentration through aerosol and then dissipate through the body to arrive at the heart (a major organ for side-effects) at a much lower concentration. The opioid receptor antagonist naloxone can actually yield completely different clinical profiles when given by different routes *in vivo*. When administered intravenously for opiate overdose, the drug gains access to the brain where it is needed. If given via the oral route it acts exclusively on bowels to treat constipation during pain therapy without affecting the central pain-reducing effects of opiates.

Naloxone

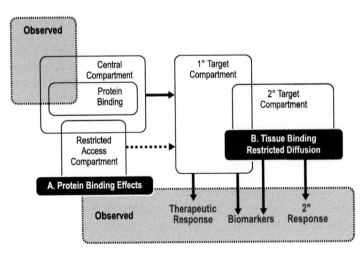

FIGURE 9.2 Shaded areas represent the experimentally accessible points of an *in vivo* experiment. Plasma samples from the central compartment can be assessed for levels of free and protein-bound drug and linked to observed effect either directly or through biomarkers.

BOX 9.5

PLASMA PROTEIN BINDING CAN OBSCURE PHARMACOKINETICS

While plasma protein binding (PPB) may not seriously alter drug development strategy (see Box 8.1), it should not be ignored when pharmacokinetic profiles of compounds and/or quantitative relationships between dose and response *in vivo* are required. The figure below shows the difference in the veracity of predictions for human clearance made through allometric scaling. When PPB is not measured and corrected for, the regression for the α_{1A}-adrenoceptor antagonist tamsulocin shows how the observed value falls considerably short of the allometric projection. This difference is greatly reduced when corrections are made for free drug concentration (data drawn from [9]).

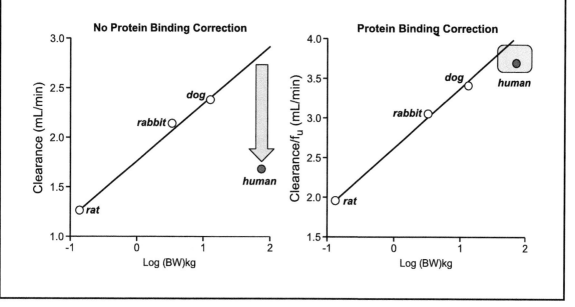

the amount of protein and concentration of drug, the dosage level at which this occurs varies. As seen in Fig. 9.3B, the observed response to a drug that is 97% protein bound occurs at concentrations considerably greater than the true free drug concentration, since only 3% of the added drug is free to produce a physiological response.

Plasma protein binding can be species-dependent; therefore it is important to quantify from actual *in vivo* samples to normalize dosing data. Figure 9.4 shows a convenient apparatus for this; plasma samples are placed into a centrifuge tube separated into compartments by a semi-permeable membrane. This allows aqueous media and dissolved free drug to pass to the bottom layer and protein (and protein-bound drug) to be retained on the membrane after centrifugation. Thus, plasma samples from *in vivo* experiments can be rapidly assessed for free drug for evaluation of true dose–response sensitivity. Shown in this

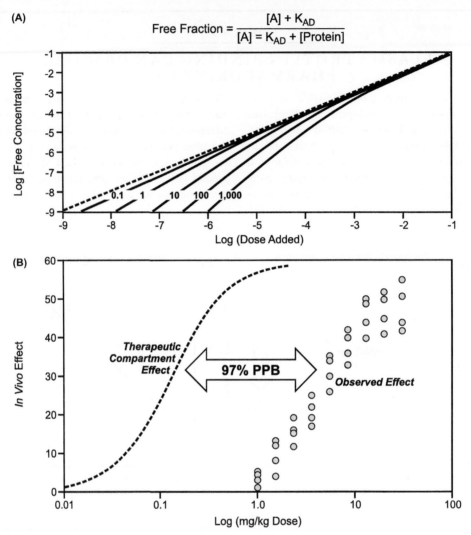

FIGURE 9.3   Plasma protein binding. (A) Ordinates reflect the level of free drug as a function of drug added to an *in vivo* system containing protein that can bind the drug. As the level of added drug increases, the binding becomes saturated and the level of free drug then equals the level of added drug. This effect is inversely proportional to the amount of protein in the system. (B) Dose–response curve of observed effect (ordinates) as a function of added drug (open circles) for a drug that is 97% protein bound. Thus, a level of 3 mg added results of only approximately 0.09 mg free drug available for response. The dotted line represents the true sensitivity of the response system to the drug.

figure is the 350% variation in plasma protein binding of the antibiotic CS-023 with species.[1]

If the therapeutic compartment (containing the target of interest for primary activity) has restricted diffusion for entry, then differences between drug levels in the central compartment and the therapeutic compartment (beyond those caused by plasma protein binding) can be further exacerbated. In such a compartment the rate at which the drug achieves

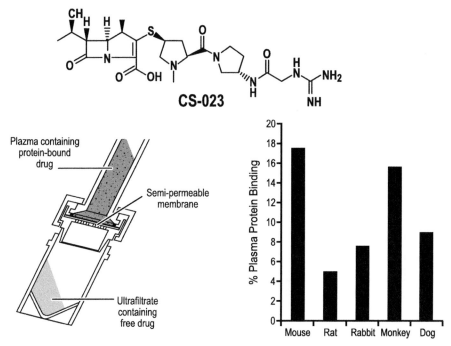

FIGURE 9.4 Apparatus in left panel allows separation of protein-bound drug (deposited on membrane) and free drug (captured in lower vessel) by centrifugation. Bar graph on right shows plasma protein binding for the antibiotic CS-023 in different animal species (data from [1]).

steady-state concentration at the biological target is given by:

$$[A_t] = (1 - e^{-(Q/V)t}) \qquad (9.1)$$

where $[A_t]$ is the concentration in the compartment at time t, the rate of diffusion is Q and the volume of the compartment is V. As in all *in vivo* systems, there is a rate of dissolution from the compartment through either degradation within the compartment or bulk diffusion out as clearance reduces the central compartment drug level. In restricted access compartments Q may be inordinately low, causing a fall in steady-state concentration into the therapeutic compartment beyond that seen in the central compartment. These are local effects and the means to measure them may not be available except through a technology amenable to detailed analysis such as imaging (see

Box 8.4). Another factor made evident from equation 9.1 is the relative volume of the therapeutic compartment; if this is large then differences in the concentration gradient (between the central (measurable) compartment and therapeutic (restricted) compartment) may be further compromised. Since the body is comprised of numerous diffusion-limited compartments, these effects constitute some of the main reasons for difficulty in equating *in vitro* drug response with the dose administered *in vivo*.

As discussed briefly in Chapter 7, another factor in evaluating *in vivo* response is the production of pharmacologically active metabolites. These must be identified so that *in vivo* response can be correctly ascribed to the parent compound or an active metabolite. For example, Fig. 9.5 shows the production of

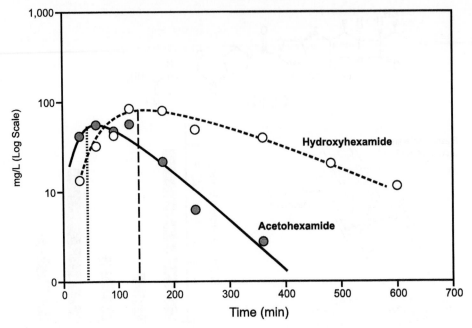

FIGURE 9.5 Production of an active metabolite from acetohexamide *in vivo*. The effects of the active metabolite are considerably more prolonged than those of the parent (data from [2]).

hydroxyhexamide from the parent acetohexamide;[2] the $t_{1/2}$ of the parent is 58 minutes while that of the metabolite is much longer ($t_{1/2} = 141$ minutes). Response is produced by both of these molecules; therefore, depending on the extent of metabolism in various species, the $t_{1/2}$ for the response could vary considerably. Table 9.1 gives a partial list of drugs that produce active metabolites *in vivo*.

WHAT CONSTITUTES DRUG RESPONSE?

Assuming that a suitable estimation can be made of the levels of active drug in the target compartment, the other variable to be considered is response. Usually, response is defined by the therapeutic endpoint for the drug. For example, a bronchodilator for asthma is aimed at relaxation of hypersensitive and constricted bronchioles to alleviate constricted breathing. Ideally, the effect of a drug *in vivo* can be visualized in real time within a time-scale that can be associated with dosage of drug. For example, aspirin given for a fever produces a fairly rapid reduction in body temperature. There are many drug responses, however, which occur only on chronic dosing (reduction in viral load in AIDS) or do not produce immediately observable effects. To monitor these types of responses, biomarkers are often used. Biomarkers in medicine furnish an indicator of the physiological or pathophysiological state of an organ that can be monitored as a surrogate for drug effectiveness. They can be direct observations (such as insulin levels, heart rate, etc.) or biochemical products of a reaction associated with a drug or pathological process (see Box 9.6). Biomarkers can be cells, molecules, genes, gene products, enzymes or

TABLE 9.1 Drugs that Form Active Metabolites through Hepatic Metabolism

Drug	Metabolite
Acetylsalicyclic acid	Salicylic acid
Amitriptyline	Nortriptyle
Carbamazepine	Carbamazepine 10,11-epoxide
Chlordiazepoxide	Desmethyl chlordiazepoxide
Codeine	Morphine
Diazepam	Desmethyldiazepam
Enalapril	Enaliprilat
Encainide	O-desmethylencainide
Fluoxetine	Norfluoxetine
Imipramine	Desipramine
Isosorbide dinitrate	Isosorbide 5-monobitrate
Meperidine	Normeperidine
Morphine	Morphine 6-glucuronide
Prazepam	Desmethyl diazepam
Prednisone	Prednisolone
Primidone	Phenobarbital
Procainamide	N-acetylprocainamide
Sulindac	Sulindac sulfide
Verapamil	Norverapamil
Zidovudine	Zidovudine triphosphate

hormones. Several biomarkers are associated specifically with disease such as serum low density cholesterol for cardiovascular disease, blood pressure for hypertension and P53 gene or matrix metalloproteinases for cancer. Figure 9.6 shows plasma drug levels of the anti-cancer drug dasatinib in immunodeficient mice implanted with K562 human chronic myeloid leukemia xenograft tumors. In this case, the tumor produces a unique biomarker in the form of BCR-ABL, a constitutively active tyrosine kinase.[3] It can be seen that the biomarker levels track drug levels, thereby linking the drug to the response. One of the most useful types of biomarkers is imaging, as in the use of rubidium chloride to evaluate perfusion of heart muscle. Imaging biomarkers tend to be more closely associated with expressed phenotype of diseases and can furnish a better association between dose and therapeutic effect. In addition, imaging is versatile, offers continuous assessments of therapy over time, can be done in animals and humans (thereby yielding translational data), and is non-invasive. Now well established, imaging is relatively simple as a method of measuring drug response (as well as pharmacokinetics; see Box 8.4). One of the most important areas for imaging as a measure of drug response is cancer where tumor size can immediately be measured after drug treatment.[4] Table 9.2 gives a partial list of common biomarkers used in medicine to assess drug effectiveness and disease state.

Considering biomarkers as indicators of effect can be speculative, i.e., there may be a number of possible biomarkers available for disease state and effectiveness of drug treatment. To evaluate these, receiver operated characteristic (ROC) curve analysis can be useful. This procedure was introduced during World War II to characterize the ability of radar operators to discern friendly versus hostile aircraft. In this procedure, a regression of the fraction of truly positive events that are correctly identified as positive (CPF) are made upon the fraction of truly negative events that are correctly identified (CNF). This is then used as a ROC curve to assess biomarkers; an example of this is shown in Fig. 9.7.

Another aspect of measuring drug response *in vivo* is the variation in the magnitude of drug response with the existing normal physiological basal tone of the system. For example, physiological heart rate is somewhat elevated as a result of the basal endogenous activity of the sympathetic nervous system. There are situations where *in vitro* testing of drugs in

BOX 9.6

BIOMARKERS: NATURE'S MESSENGERS FOR PHYSIOLOGICAL STATE

Reduction in blood flow to the heart (through blockage of one or more blood vessels) in conditions such as unstable angina or heart attack can cause chest pain, shortness of breath, nausea, sweating and dizziness. If prolonged, this condition can lead to damage to the heart muscle in the form of an infarction and thus can be life-threatening. There are cases where myocardial infarctions may be "silent" or clinically unrecognized and in these cases, a biomarker can be a valuable indication of possible cardiac damage. The most reliable biomarker used by physicians for detection of cardiac damage from such episodes is the detection of troponins in the blood. Although troponins exist in other cell types, cardiac troponin I is unique and thus can be specifically identified. This makes troponin I the only specific biomarker for cardiac muscle. Levels rise 4 to 6 hours after infarction and may remain elevated for up to 7 days, thereby leaving a lasting record of the event.

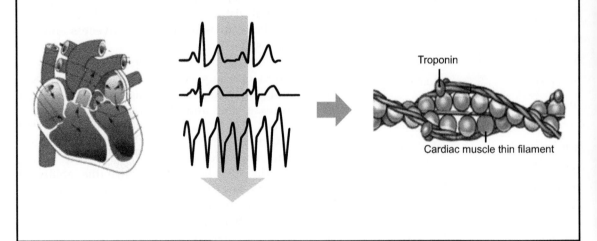

systems devoid of basal activation may yield data different to that observed *in vivo* because of this factor. The most obvious cases occur for weak partial agonists. Figure 9.8 shows how a partial agonist may increase physiological activity in conditions of low physiological tone and decrease activity under conditions of high physiological tone.

Finally, the body has mechanisms to counter imbalance and attain stability; some of these are neuronal reflexes and it is difficult to predict drug effect on these processes from *in vitro* experiments. Reflexes can be important determinants of drug utility; for example, unabated hypotension through blockade of pressor α-adrenoceptor activation robs the patient of reflexes to counter postural hypotension; this can lead to fainting when patients stand. Box 9.7 shows a reflex mechanism that produces a favorable drug effect.

As discussed in Chapter 3 (see Figs 3.1, 3.2) tissue-related factors can control sensitivity to

(A)

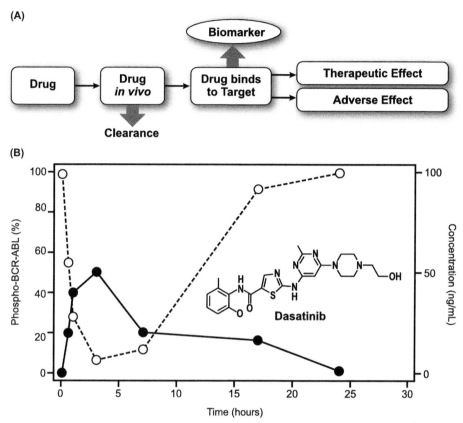

FIGURE 9.6 Biomarkers. (A) Schematic diagram of the production of a biomarker produced by a system in direct response to the action of a drug. (B) Biomarker for cancer (BCR-ABL, a constitutively active tyrosine kinase produced by the tumor) shown as open circles (dotted line) as a function of time. Filled circles show central compartment concentrations of an antitumor drug dasatinib (drawn from [3]).

hormones, transmitters and synthetic agonists. Specifically, the amount of target in the cell (e.g., densities of cell surface receptors) and how efficiently the target is coupled to cellular response mechanisms can produce a wide range of sensitivities. The Black–Leff operational model (see Chapter 3) can be used to relate the power of agonists to activate a given organ system; this can be done *in vitro* in a test system. Figure 9.9A shows the *in vitro* dose–response curves to two agonists, a standard and a test compound. From this type of analysis, the relative efficacy (relative τ values)

and relative affinities for the target can be measured. If a dose–response curve to the standard agonist is available *in vivo*, then the change in sensitivity of the *in vitro* test system versus the *in vivo* therapeutic system can be made through quantification of the change in τ for the standard agonist. Under these circumstances, the relative power of the test agonist can then be assessed. This is shown in Fig. 9.9B where it can be seen that the *in vivo* system is considerably less sensitive than the *in vitro* system. The change in sensitivity from the *in vitro* to the *in vivo* system is then applied

TABLE 9.2   Some Common Biomarkers

Biomarker	Denotes
• Prostate specific antigen (PSA)	Prostate cancer
• Human papilloma virus	Environmental exposure to toxic substances
• ↑Dimethylarginine	Cardiovascular disease
• ↑Insulin levels	Diabetes
• C-reactive protein (CRP)	Inflammation; can be indicator of effectiveness of anti-inflammatory therapy
• ↑Cholesterol	Cardiovascular disease
• ↑Creatinine kinase	Biomarker of muscle damage
• ↑Fibrinogen in venous blood	Cardiovascular disease; also an acute phase protein in inflammation

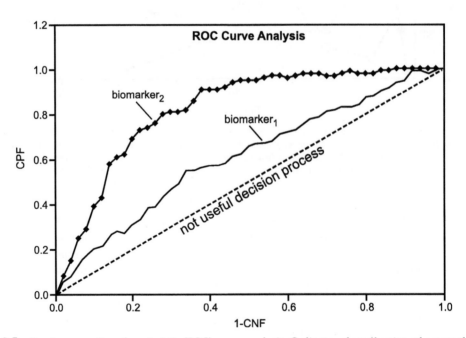

FIGURE 9.7   Receiver operating characteristic (ROC) curve analysis. Ordinate values (fraction of events that are correctly correlated with biomarker; CPF) plotted as a regression on 1 − the fraction of negative events that are correctly identified with the biomarker (1 − CNF). The dotted straight line indicates random chance (50–50% chance of prediction with biomarker). Skewed lines in the top left quadrant reflect increasing ability of the test to correctly predict outcomes. This particular curve shows that biomarker$_2$ is a better predictor of the event than biomarker$_1$.

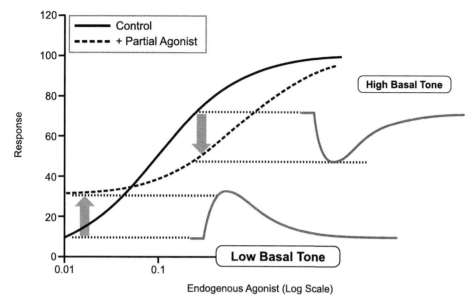

FIGURE 9.8 Dose–response curves to an endogenous full agonist *in vivo* in the presence and absence of a single concentration of partial agonist. Solid line represents system response to the full agonist in the absence of partial agonist. Dotted line shows the response to the full agonist in the presence of a concentration of partial agonist. In conditions of low basal tone (low concentrations of endogenous full agonist), the partial agonist will produce stimulation. Under conditions of high endogenous basal tone (higher ambient concentration of endogenous full agonist), the partial agonist will produce antagonism.

to the test agonist (see Fig. 3.6) for prediction of the sensitivity of the *in vivo* system to the test agonist. As shown in Fig. 9.9C, the relative efficacy of the test to standard agonist coupled with the reduction in sensitivity of the *in vivo* system (compared to the *in vitro* system) predicts that little, if any, response will be observed in the *in vivo* system to the test agonist. These types of predictions can be very useful in assessing *in vivo* responses (or lack of responses) to agonists.

THE IMPORTANCE OF KINETICS
IN VIVO

In vitro experimentation to optimize drug activity emphasizes intensity of effect (i.e.,

potency, efficacy, etc.). However, for open (*in vivo*) systems, the kinetics of effects are equally, and sometimes more, important. Therefore, the duration of effect becomes a critical variable in the assessment of drug activity. If the duration is linked to elimination pharmacokinetics, then assuming that final elimination can be described by a single compartment after drug distribution throughout the body, concentration with time is given by:

$$[C]_t = (Dose/V_d)e^{-kt} \qquad (9.2)$$

where V_d is the volume of distribution, k is an elimination rate constant and t is time. Defining $t_{duration}$ as the time the concentration is above an arbitrary therapeutically defined

BOX 9.7

REFLEXES BECOME IMPORTANT TO *IN VIVO* DRUG ACTIVITY

β-adrenoceptor agonists produce increased force of contraction (measured as the rate of rise of left ventricular pressure, Δdp/dt); theoretically this effect could be of benefit in congestive heart failure as, in this disease, cardiac contractility is reduced and considerable congestion occurs due to inefficient left ventricular emptying. A major limitation to the use of β-agonists is the fact that they also promote debilitating increases in heart rate; this is shown for isoproterenol where increases in contractility (ΔdP/dt40) are accompanied by increased heart rate. The same problematic heart rate effect is not seen with the β-agonist Dobutamine (panel on right). This is because Dobutamine posseses a low level of α-adrenoceptor activation to slightly elevate vascular tone. This, in turn, activates the baroreceptor reflex to repress increases in heart rate. The slight activation of the baroreceptor reflex allows Dobutamine to be a limited use inotropic drug in humans; this effect is only seen *in vivo* (data from [10]).

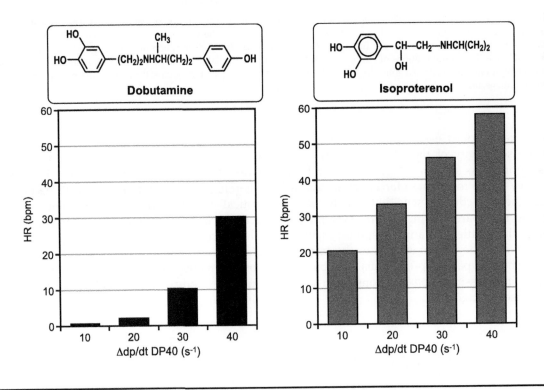

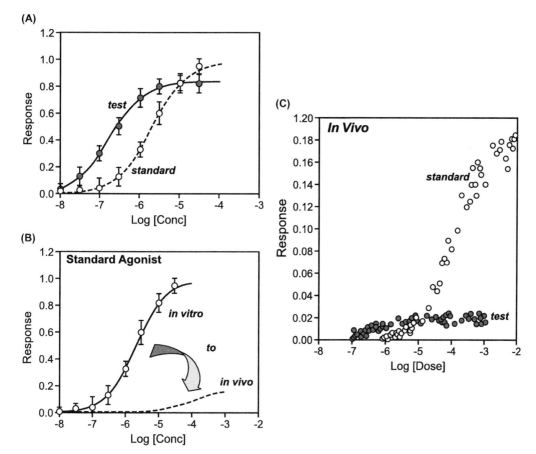

FIGURE 9.9 Application of the Black–Leff operational model of agonism (Chapter 3) for the prediction of agonist response *in vivo*. (A) Effects of a standard and test agonist in an *in vitro* test system. These data furnish estimates of the relative efficacy (τ values) and affinities of the agonists. (B) Measure of the change in sensitivity from the *in vitro* system to the *in vivo* system for the standard agonist. This gives an estimate of the change in τ value for the standard agonist in going from the *in vitro* to the *in vivo* system. (C) The change in τ value for the standard agonist is applied to the test agonist (applied to the relative τ value determined *in vitro*) to predict the dose–response curve to the test agonist *in vivo*. It can be seen from this case that the relative τ values determined in Panel (A) predict that essentially no agonism to the test agonist will be seen *in vivo*.

minimal level (C_{min}), and setting $k = 0.693$ $(t_{1/2})^{-1}$, equation 9.2 defines the duration of action as:

$$t_{duration} = 1.44\ t_{1/2}(\ln[Dose] - (V_d \bullet C_{min}))\quad(9.3)$$

Under these circumstances, the duration of action is proportional to the $t_{1/2}$ for drug elimination if effect is linked to pharmacokinetics. The various procedures described in Chapter 7 and Chapter 8 can be used to estimate $t_{1/2}$ and a measure of duration of drug action can be made.

Since drug response is linked to kinetics in open systems, observed potencies can be affected by the time following dosage that the

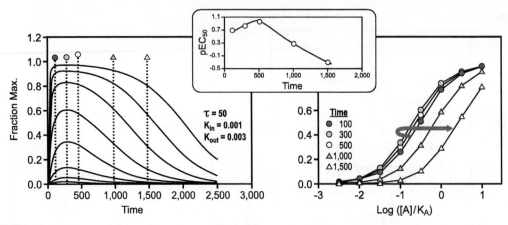

FIGURE 9.10   Influence of the analysis of agonism, at different time-points, on the observed potency of the agonist. It can be seen that the time-point at which the agonism is measured controls the location of the dose–response curve to the agonist along the drug concentration axis, i.e., potency is a function of time in an open system. Inset shows pEC$_{50}$ of the agonist with time.

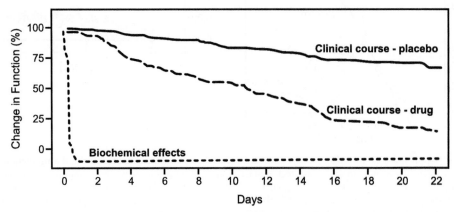

FIGURE 9.11   Effect of an antidepressant on clinical depression with time. For antidepressant drugs that are inhibitors of monamine transport (dopamine, serotonin, norepinephrine), a rapid increase in the synaptic cleft concentration of neurotransmitter is observed within 1 to 2 days. The measurable improvement in subjective indices of depression, however, requires a much longer time to become evident. Thus there is a discontinuity between the biochemical effect and the therapeutic effect.

measurements are taken. Figure 9.10 shows a dose–response curve to an agonist as a function of time; it can be seen from this figure that the time at which response is measured can have important effects on the reported potency of the agonist *in vivo*. There also can actually be large discrepancies between clinically effective responses to drugs and the initial biochemical events that trigger them. Figure 9.11 shows the time course for alleviation of the symptoms of depression as a function of treatment with a monoamine uptake inhibitor. While the fairly rapidly observed biochemical event (increased neurotransmitter present in the synaptic cleft)

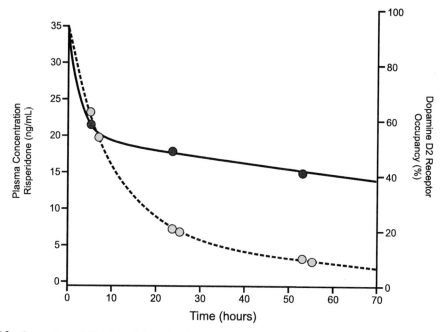

FIGURE 9.12 Separation of kinetics of drug level and drug target occupancy of dopamine D2 receptors by risperidone. Filled circles show the time course of dopamine receptor occupancy measured in human brain *in vivo* through imaging; this process has a $t_{1/2}$ of 80.2 hours. Open gray circles show the plasma concentrations of risperidone; $t_{1/2} = 17.8$ hours (drawn from [6]).

coincides with the biochemical mechanism of the drug, it takes a considerable length of time for the system to remodel itself as a result of this biochemical effect to finally produce the therapeutic effect. These are extreme discontinuities between the initiation of the pharmacologic effect and the eventual return to normal physiology. Similar effects are seen in cancer chemotherapy where complete elimination of tumors may require prolonged biochemical treatment.

There are a number of common circumstances where central compartment pharmacokinetics is not the only consideration in defining duration of drug effect *in vivo*. For instance, if the therapeutic target resides in a diffusion-restricted compartment, then efflux to and from this compartment may be slower than it is from the central compartment, and duration may be longer than that predicted from

central compartment pharmacokinetics. In a restricted compartment, drug that has diffused from the target may rebind due to confined volume effects or binding to high affinity "exosites" within the compartment.[5] These effects are difficult to predict reliably although imaging of distinct regions may be an option. Figure 9.12 shows how reversal of the brain dopamine D2 receptor occupancy of the antipsychotic drug risperidone with time (as observed through imaging) is considerably slower than the clearance of the drug from the central compartment. Specifically, the $t_{1/2}$ for clearance from the central compartment is 17.8 hours while the $t_{1/2}$ for offset from receptors in the brain is 80.2 hours.[6]

One mechanism to predict the duration of effect that can be evaluated *in vitro* is the kinetics of binding of the molecule to the biological target. The kinetics of receptor dissociation can be extremely important to *in vivo* target coverage (a term encompassing dissociation of the drug from the target with time *in vivo*). If the offset of the antagonist from the receptor is slow, then the antagonism can far outlast the presence of the antagonist in the receptor compartment. The kinetics of offset from the receptor once the antagonist is bound is given by:

$$\rho_{t-off} = \rho_e e^{-k_2 t} \qquad (9.4)$$

The potency of the antagonist is given by the equilibrium dissociation constant of the antagonist–receptor complex defined as the ratio $K_B = k_2/k_1$. For example, Fig. 9.13 shows association and dissociation curves for two antihistamines; diphenhydramine has a potency of 31.5 nM and triprolidine has a potency of 3.14 nM. While these antagonists differ in potency, they also differ widely in kinetics. The rate of dissociation (from the receptor) of diphenhydramine is 8.1 times the rate of dissociation of triprolidine, causing the antagonism by diphenhydramine to be much more transient than an equiactive dose of triprolidine in

an open system. Differences in dissociation kinetics need not necessarily be obvious from antagonist potency. Since a near infinite range of k_2 and k_1 values can yield the same K_B, it can be seen that antagonists of identical potencies can have a wide range of onset and offset kinetics. For example, a nanomolar potency antagonist (i.e., $K_B = 10^{-9}$ M) can have a rate of onset of 5×10^5 s^{-1} mol^{-1} and a rate of offset of 5×10^{-4} s^{-1} (consider this a "rapid" offset antagonist) or a rate of onset of 10^5 s^{-1} mol^{-1} and offset of 10^{-4} s^{-1} ("slow" offset). While these molecules are equipotent in a closed system at equilibrium (i.e., in an *in vitro* assay), they will give widely different temporal target coverage *in vivo*. Specifically, the "slow" antagonist will give a much longer coverage of the receptor than the "fast" antagonist. Box 9.8 shows how the serotonin antagonists altanserin and ritanserin, which are similar in potency, have vastly different target coverage capabilities.

Dissociation kinetics of antagonists can become very important in light of the fact that the exposure of the target to the antagonist *in vivo*

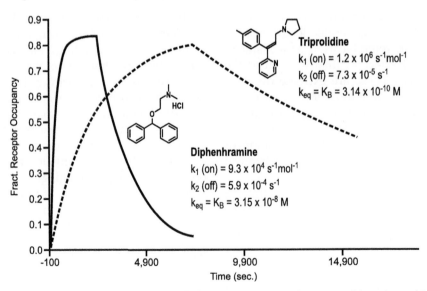

FIGURE 9.13 Graph of theoretical association and dissociation patterns for two antihistamines of known potency. Addition of the antagonist leads to an increasing receptor occupancy until a plateau is reached, while washing causes reversal of occupancy with antagonist dissociation. Diphenhydramine is a rapidly acting antagonist while triprolidine is slow.

BOX 9.8

TARGET RESIDENCY MAY BE MORE IMPORTANT THAN POTENCY

The absolute potency of receptor antagonists is an important parameter since it is directly linked to the amount of drug that must be present in the target compartment to produce an antagonist effect. However, since the body is an open system, the concentration of drug varies with time; therefore the target is exposed to a "wave" of drug for a certain period and then the pool is removed from the target compartment. Therefore, the amount of time it takes for the antagonist to dissociate from the receptor becomes an integral factor in the amount of

time the antagonist can produce target coverage (i.e., be associated with the target to cause a therapeutic effect). This dissociation time can be somewhat different from the potency, thus it becomes another factor in the antagonist profile. The serotonin antagonists altanserin and ritanserin have relatively similar potencies (altanserin $pK_B = 9.37$ and ritanserin $pK_B = 9.05$) but the $t_{1/2}$ for dissociation of ritanserin is more than 10 times greater. This would produce considerably better target coverage *in vivo* (data from [11]).

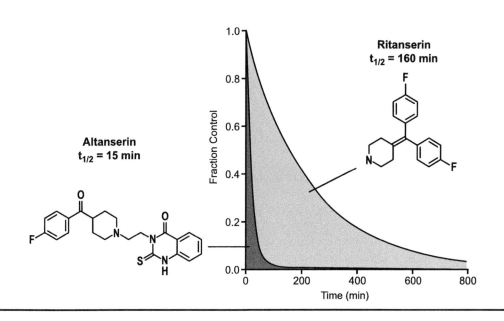

is transient. If dissociation kinetics are slow then a transient exposure of target to antagonist may "load" the system and antagonism may persist long after the receptor compartment is free of antagonist. Figure 9.14 shows the receptor

occupancy for antagonists of varying offset kinetics after a transient exposure of antagonist *in vivo*. It can be seen that slow rates of offset can cause persistent receptor occupancy by the antagonist that do not follow the pharmacokinetics of

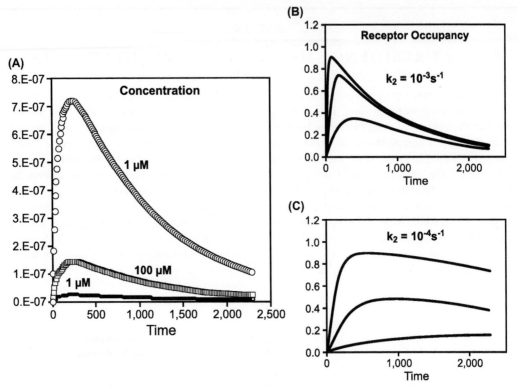

FIGURE 9.14   Correspondence between antagonist target coverage and antagonist absorption. Panel (A) shows the absorption and pharmacokinetics for an antagonist. Panel (B) shows the corresponding receptor occupancy with time for the antagonist if it has a rapid dissociation ($k_2 = 10^{-3}$ s^{-1}). Panel (C): Receptor coverage with time if the same antagonist had a much slower rate of dissociation ($1/10 \times$ to yield $k_2 = 10^{-4}$ s^{-1}).

antagonist concentration in the receptor compartment.

Very slow antagonist dissociation can be useful in producing long periods of target coverage, even after the molecule has been cleared from the body. Figure 9.15A shows dissociation curves for the chemokine CCL3 and three allosteric HIV-1 entry inhibitors from the therapeutic target, namely the CCR5 chemokine receptor. It can be seen that the $t_{1/2}$ values for aplaviroc, maraviroc and Sch-C are considerably longer than 24 hours.[7] Figure 9.15B shows a simulated target coverage for aplaviroc in contrast to plasma concentration. It can be seen that the association with the target continues long after aplaviroc has been

cleared. For aplaviroc, the slow dissociation kinetics allows it to be a once-per-day treatment even though the pharmacokinetics of concentration in the plasma does not support that regimen of dosing. In this case, the target coverage was assessed by noting that lymphocytes derived from patients 24 hours after treatment still failed to be infected by HIV-1, indicating that aplaviroc is still bound to CCR5 at that time. Dissociation between the pharmacokinetic concentration of drugs in the central compartment and their target coverage *in vivo* offers a tool to pharmacologists for the improvement of *in vivo* therapy. Due to this fact, the *in vitro* measurement of drug–target dissociation rate becomes an important part of

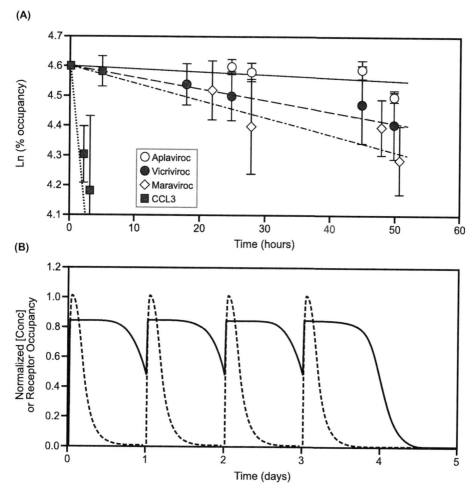

FIGURE 9.15 Antagonist dissociation kinetics and target coverage. (A) Dissociation of allosteric HIV-1 entry inhibitors from CCR5 receptors. The $t_{1/2}$ values range from being fairly rapid ($t_{1/2}$ = 2.7 hours for CCL3) to increasingly prolonged ($t_{1/2}$ = 53 hours (Sch-C), 192 hours (maraviroc) and >200 hours (aplaviroc)) (data from [7]). (B) Simulated target coverage (solid line) and central compartment levels of aplaviroc (dotted line) when aplaviroc is given every 24 hours.

the characterization of the activity of drugs, as much as the measurement of steady-state equilibrium measures of potency and efficacy.

SUMMARY

- The ultimate therapeutic value of a molecule is determined by its effect *in vivo*;

factors such as plasma protein binding, endogenous physiological tone and reflexes can obscure the relationship between free drug concentration and observed effect.
- The response to a drug may be observed directly or through a surrogate such as a biochemical biomarker. In addition, there may be temporal dissociation between the actual biochemical events initiated by the

drug and the eventual lasting therapeutic response.

- The Black–Leff operational model (Chapter 3) can be very useful in translating *in vitro* agonist effect into predicted effects *in vivo*.
- Since *in vivo* systems are open systems, response must be linked with time of exposure to drug.
- The kinetics of drug movement within the body is immensely important to the *in vivo* activity of drugs either through restricted diffusion to and from the compartments containing the therapeutic target or through the actual rate of dissociation of the drug from the target itself.
- The rate of drug-target dissociation can greatly augment otherwise rapid and inadequate pharmacokinetics for therapy.
- It is important to quantify the rate of drug–target dissociation as an integral part of the profile of a given drug candidate (in addition to potency and efficacy).

QUESTIONS

9.1 An agonist for β-adrenoceptors has excellent permeation properties *in vivo* and a low value for clearance. In addition, this compound is extremely potent in cell culture cyclic AMP studies *in vitro* ($pEC_{50} = 8.1$). In spite of this profile, the *in vivo* profile is disappointing and little bronchodilation was observed. What could be happening?

9.2 An antitumor compound was active against xenograft tumors in mice but proved to be disappointing in humans. Analysis of total compound showed plasma levels to be comparable, eliminating differences in pharmacokinetics to be the cause. What else could be occurring?

9.3 Two anticholinergic antagonists of comparable potency *in vitro* are tested for hyperactive urinary bladder *in vivo*. One shows clearly superior effects over the other even though both have comparable levels of clearance and plasma protein binding. What additional experiments would be useful to examine this problem?

9.4 A β₂-adrenoceptor agonist for alleviation of airway constriction in asthma is found to be six-fold more potent in relaxing constricted airway muscle than in producing harmful tachycardia in experiments done *in vitro*. While this ratio is not considered high and suggests that the compound would have dangerous cardiovascular effects, it is still worth testing *in vivo*. Why?

References

[1] T. Shibayama, Y. Matsushita, A. Kurihara, T. Hirota, T. Ikeda, Prediction of pharmacokinetics of CS-023 (RO4908463), a novel parenteral carbapenemantibiotic, in humans using animal data, Xenobiotica 37 (2007) 91–102.

[2] J.A. Galloway, R.E. McMahon, H.W. Culp, F.J. Marshall, E.C. Young, Metabolism, blood levels and rate of excretion of acetohexamide in human subjects, Diabetes 16 (1967) 118–127.

[3] F.R. Luo, Z. Yang, A. Camuso, R. Smykla, K. McGlinchey, K. Fager, et al., Dasatinib (BMS-354825) pharmacokinetics and pharmacodynamic biomarkers in animal models predict optimal clinical exposure, Clin. Canc. Res. 12 (2006) 7180–7186.

[4] M. Rudin, R. Weissleder, Molecular imaging in drug discovery and development, Nature Rev. Drug Disc. 2 (2003) 123–131.

[5] G. Vauquelin, S.J. Charlton, Long-lasting target binding and rebinding as mechanisms to prolong in vivo drug action, Br. J. Pharmacol. 161 (2010) 488–508.

[6] A. Takano, T. Suhara, Y. Ikoma, F. Tasuno, J. Maeda, T. Ichimiya, et al., Estimation of the time-course of dopamine D2 receptor occupancy in living human brain from plasma pharmacokinetics of antipsychotics, Int. J. Neuropsychopharmacol. 7 (2004) 19–26.

[7] C. Watson, S. Jenkinson, W. Kazmierski, T.P. Kenakin, The CCR5 receptor-based mechanism of action of 873140, a potent allosteric non-competitive HIV entry-inhibitor, Mol. Pharmacol. 67 (2005) 1268–1282.

[8] S. Carpenter, M. Rigaud, M. Barile, T.J. Priest, L. Perez, J.B. Ferguson, An interlinear transliteration and English translation of portions of The Ebers Papryus possibly having to do with diabetes mellitus, Bard College, Annandale-on-Hudson, NY, 1998.

[9] E. Van Hoogdalem, Y. Soeishi, H. Matsushima, S. Higuchi, Disposition of the selective α1A-adrenoceptor antagonist tamsulosin in humans: Comparison with data from interspecies scaling, J. Pharm. Sci. 86 (1997) 1156–1161.

[10] T.P. Kenakin, S.F. Johnson, The importance of α-adrenoceptor agonist activity of dobutamine to inotropic selectivity in the anaesthetized cat, Eur. J. Pharmacol. 111 (1985) 347–354.

[11] J.E. Leysen, W. Gommeren, Drug-receptor dissociation time, new tool for drug research: Receptor binding affinity and drug-receptor dissociation profiles of serotonin-S2, dopamine D2 and histamine H1 antagonists and opiates, Drug. Dev. Res. 8 (1986) 119–131.

10

Safety Pharmacology

By the end of this chapter the reader will be aware of the breadth of assays and testing procedures available to assess the safety of a new drug entity. In addition, readers will be able to identify rapid *in vitro* tests that can detect serious toxicity in molecules at a very early stage. Finally, this chapter should yield an understanding of toxicity due to elevated drug exposure (intrinsic toxicity) versus that due to stochastic opportunity (idiosyncratic toxicity) showing how the latter is difficult to predict in drug testing and thus poses a serious risk in the drug development process.

INTRODUCTION

In addition to having primary activity and being able to enter the body, access the appropriate tissue and have sufficient target presence to achieve therapeutic utility, a drug must cause no harm to the host. Therefore, the third important structure—activity relationship that must be explored for a drug is safety pharmacology. The human body is a finely tuned symphony of biochemical reactions and physiological functions, and miscues can cause the system to go awry. It is unrealistic to suppose that extreme amounts of almost any substance won't eventually cause harm; as put by Paracelsus (1493–1541):

> "... all things are poison and nothing is without poison. Solely the dose determines that a thing is not poison ..."

The concept of "safety" can also be relative. As pointed out in the discussion of target validation in Chapter 1, one of the criteria in the choice of a favorable target for an antagonist is that the knockout mouse (genetically altered such that the target is not expressed in tissues) is healthy, i.e., the organism can do without the target. Thus it was observed that CCR5 knockout mice (lacking the CCR5 receptor) were healthy, thereby indicating that the CCR5 receptor is redundant and not required for life. While this spurred on pursuit of CCR5 as a target for HIV-1-mediated AIDS infection, the idea that CCR5 is redundant and not required for health was later shown to be simplistic. In this case, there is a human counterpart to the CCR5 knockout mouse, namely a population of people possessing a Δ32 CCR5 deletion in the receptor that causes it not to be expressed on the cell surface; in essence, human equivalent "knockouts." These people appeared to have normal health; however, as data accumulated this concept of "healthy" began to be questioned. Specifically, it had been shown that Δ32 subjects have a higher than average incidence of health abnormalities (i.e., greater incidence of liver disease and schlerosing cholangitis,[1] risk of death in Nile Virus disease,[2] greater mortality after liver transplantation,[3] mild immunodeficiency[4]). The point of these data for this chapter is to suggest that chemical intervention into *any* physiological function almost necessarily brings with it a risk of imbalance and consequent risk of harm. Therefore, it is a defensible statement to suggest that all drugs, if given in sufficient dosage, may have harmful side-effects and pharmacological safety is simply a matter of relative benefit to risk of harm. This chapter will consider this benefit-to-risk ratio for drugs.

NEW TERMINOLOGY

The following new terms will be introduced in this chapter:

- **Carcinogenesis**: The creation of cancer where normal cells are transformed into cancer cells
- **Cytotoxicity**: The quality of being toxic to cells to detrimentally affect cell metabolism, function, growth and to subsequently induce damage.
- **Idiosyncratic toxicity**: Toxic effects due to stochastic probability occurring when a combination of favorable conditions coalesce.

- **Intrinsic toxicity**: Toxicity due to elevation of dosage above a threshold for toxicity, i.e., it is observed whenever this dosage is exceeded.
- **MTD**: Maximum tolerated dose – applies to long-term studies and refers to the largest dose that causes no obvious signs of ill health.
- **Mutagenesis**: Induction of genetic change in a cell through alteration of cell genetic material (usually DNA).
- **NOAEL**: No observed adverse effect level – the largest dose causing no observed toxicity or undesirable physiological effect.
- **NOEL**: No observed effect level – the threshold for producing a pharmacologic or toxic effect.
- **NTEL**: No toxic effect level – the largest dose in most sensitive species that produces no toxic effect.

SAFETY VERSUS TOXICITY

Drug safety is often discussed in terms of "toxicology" when it is really more appropriate to focus on the term safety, defined as "the condition of being safe from undergoing ... hurt, injury." Presupposing that a drug will cause harm if used inappropriately or in too high a dose, the aim is to define the conditions whereby a drug can be used effectively to heal with minimal risk of toxicity (defined as "containing or being a poisonous material ... capable of causing death or serious debillitation"). For example, the drug theophylline is used intravenously in emergency rooms for acute bronchoconstriction in children. While a serum concentration of $15 \, \mu g/mL$ produces life-saving bronchodilation, $25 \, \mu g/mL$ causes mild side-effects which become potentially serious at $35 \, \mu g/mL$ and severe at $42 \, \mu g/mL$. Thus, less than a three-fold increase in serum plasma levels can lead to toxicity. The key to theophylline's value is the fact that it is used in a strictly controlled setting (intravenous administration under a physician's supervision with constant surveillance). In this case, the "safety" of theophylline is an extremely qualified parameter.

There are categories of toxicity based on mechanism:

- **Undesired but expected effects**: These result from the primary pharmacology of the drug occurring by the therapeutic mechanism but in tissues other than the primary therapeutic organ. These usually cannot be avoided. Examples of this type of toxicity are digital tremor with β_2-adrenoceptor bronchodilators. Since β_2-adrenoceptors mediate bronchodilation and unwanted response (digital tremor), any such agonist will produce both effects. Restricted route of administration (aerosol) is used to minimize these side-effects.
- **Desired excessive effects**: These result from the primary pharmacology of the drug

acting on the therapeutic organ. An example of this is insulin-induced hypoglycemic reaction. These also cannot be avoided and come with excessive dose.

- **Undesired unexpected effects**: These occur by mechanisms different from the primary therapeutic mechanism of action of the drug. An example of this is the dry mouth coming from antimuscarinic effects of antihistamines such as diphenhydramine.
- **Poorly predictable effects**: These are the most problematic in that they are difficult to detect. They consist of drug allergies, idiosyncratic effects, mutagenesis, carcinogenesis and drug dependency.

There are other classifications of toxicity used such as the Type A to E listing of adverse drug reactions (see Box 10.1).

BOX 10.1

A CLASSIFICATION SYSTEM FOR ADVERSE REACTIONS

An adverse drug reaction (event) (ADR) can be defined as any undesired, noxious or unintended event occurring from a normal dosage (used for prophylaxis, diagnosis or treatment) of the drug. The Federal Drug Administration regards any outcome leading to death, risk of death, hospitalization, disability or required intervention to prevent permanent impairment or damage as adverse; these account for approximately 5% of all hospital admissions per year. Treatment failure, intentional or accidental overdose are not considered ADRs. Below is one classification of ADRs based on drug mechanism of action (data from [13]).

Mechanistic Classifications of Adverse Drug Reactions		
Classification	**Characteristics**	**Example**
Type A	• Result of Pharmacology of the Drug Target type	• High levels of anticoagulants lead to hemmorhage
Type B	• Idiosynchratic reaction and/or activation of secondary target	• Fenfluramine activation of cardiac 5-HT2B receptors
Type C	• Chemically mediated, oxidative stress, phospholipidosis, haemolysis	• Acetaminophen (paracetamol) hepatotoxicity
Type D	• Delayed after chronic treatment/cancers	• Fetal hydantoin syndrome with phenytoin
Type E	• End of treatment (withdrawal)	• Seizures after sudden withdrawal of phenytoin

SAFETY PHARMACOLOGY

There is a basic difference between safety assessment and determining primary drug efficacy. In the latter, researchers know what to look for; in safety assessment they do not. A hazard cannot be characterized until it is identified. Therefore, safety pharmacology involves the dual tasks of hazard identification and risk assessment. Hazard identification basically examines the profile of a drug and analyzes the potential harmful effects that can, and do, occur. Risk assessment then quantifies the probability that they will occur during clinical or accidental exposure. From this point other analyses are done to yield possible dose–response relationships for these effects. This involves issues such as reversibility and determination of NOAEL (no observed adverse effect level; see Chapter 8) and parameters for clinical monitoring. Other features of these analyses include examination of physical risk factors (age, gender, susceptible patient populations), environmental risk factors (conditions present that may enhance toxicity/pharmacological interactions) and genetic risk factors (genetic determinant for susceptibility to toxicity, known gene polymorphisms).

Safety assessment of drugs is an extremely important endeavor in that if a hazard is not identified, patients may be harmed. Moreover, in the drug development process, resources increase exponentially as candidate molecules reach the end of the development process; to reduce expenditure of large resources, candidates that will not be successful due to toxicity must be identified as soon as possible (see Box 10.2). As safety testing begins, a number of lines of investigation are initiated (see Table 10.1):

- **Safety pharmacology**: Detection of undesirable pharmacodynamic effects on specific organ systems. Some of these tests are simple *in vitro* experiments that can be done very early on in the development process much like *in vitro* ADME studies (CaCo-2, hepatic enzymes; *vide infra*).
- **Genetic toxicity**: Examination of possible gene mutation and chromosomal damage.
- **Single/repeat dosing studies**: Detailed examination of target toxicity and local tolerance.
- **Reproductive toxicity**: Effects on embryo-fetal development, fertility, parturition, post-natal development.
- **Carcinogenicity**: Risk of development of tumors.
- **Special studies**: Immunotoxicology, phototoxicology, environmental health and safety.

A major tool in these endeavors is the repeat dosing study. In this procedure the goal is to develop an understanding between exposure to drug and observed untoward effects, and also to assess the potential for reversibility. Response can be directly observed or the study may seek to find biomarkers for effects. The overall aim is to assess organ toxicity and safety associated with repeat dosing to predict risk in humans; the object is to specifically define the NOEL (no observed effect level), MTD (maximal tolerated dose) and NOAEL (no observed adverse effect level). The first step in this process is to achieve high exposures of systems to the drug *in vivo*. For this, pharmacokinetic effects may need to be observed at doses extended far beyond what is required therapeutically, i.e., dosing must continue (and exposure be increased) until adverse effects are detected. [5] Therefore, cases of limited exposure due to solubility (see Chapter 8 for discussion of solubility limitation for exposure to the hepatoprotective agent YH439) can be problematic. In these cases extended exposure protocols may be required which may not be applicable to therapeutic dosing. Figure 10.1 shows the effects of some solvents used for administration of experimental candidate molecules to optimize solubility and ultimately, exposure.

BOX 10.2

COSTLY DISCOVERIES

A prospective drug has incurred nearly 90% of its cost of discovery and development by the time it is in Phase III testing. Therefore it is of paramount importance that an unsuitable molecule be eliminated from development before costs rise to this level. However, even more devastating is the discovery of serious toxicity after a drug has been approved and is on the market. Below are four examples of drugs that demonstrated rare but extremely serious toxicity after marketing, causing them to be withdrawn from the market.

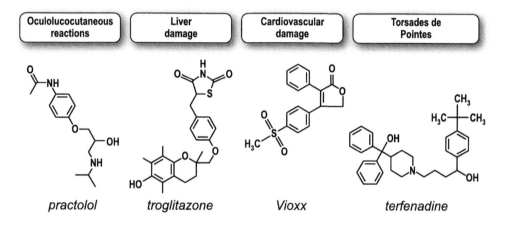

| Oculolucocutaneous reactions | Liver damage | Cardiovascular damage | Torsades de Pointes |

practolol   *troglitazone*   *Vioxx*   *terfenadine*

TABLE 10.1   Safety Pharmacology Testing During Different Stages of Drug Development

Development Phase	Safety Activity
Lead to candidate	• Acute toxicology • hERG • Ames test/cytotoxicity • Early safety prediction • 2° receptors
Candidate selection to first human dose	• Genotoxicity • Safety pharmacology dose ranging • 14–28 day toxicology studies
Patient phase 2a/2b studies	• 3/6/9/12 month toxicology studies • Reproductive toxicology studies • Immunotoxicology studies
Phase 3 clinical studies	• Carcinogenesis • Reproductive toxicology

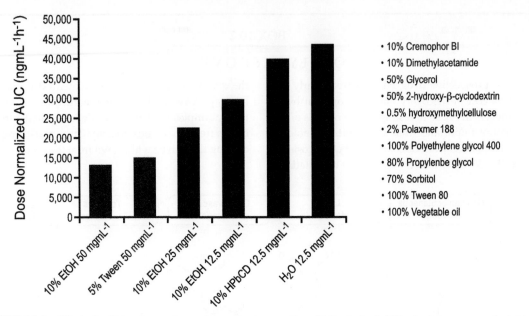

- 10% Cremophor Bl
- 10% Dimethylacetamide
- 50% Glycerol
- 50% 2-hydroxy-β-cyclodextrin
- 0.5% hydroxymethylcellulose
- 2% Polaxmer 188
- 100% Polyethylene glycol 400
- 80% Propylenbe glycol
- 70% Sorbitol
- 100% Tween 80
- 100% Vegetable oil

FIGURE 10.1 Effect of using various solvents for a new drug entity with limited solubility for intravenous administration to Cynomolgus monkeys. It can be seen that a 300% increase in exposure can be achieved through judicious use of solvent (data from [11]). A list of solvents used to increase drug exposure *in vivo* is shown in the right panel.

An element of perspective should also be used in assessing risk to high exposures. The sweetener saccharin has been used since the 1800s but was only subjected to rigorous safety testing in the 1970s. In these tests it was linked to bladder cancer in rats and subsequently recalled from the market. It was later recognized that the doses where this occurred would have required a human to ingest grams of saccharin every day from birth until 80 years of age. Moreover, the effect was *unique to rats* since there was a characteristic combination of high urine pH, level of calcium phosphate and a special protein in rat urine to cause microcrystallization of these doses of saccaharin. These eventually caused damage to the lining of the bladder where, over time, active production of cells to repair the damage leads to tumor formation. The salient points for the assessment of the safety of saccharin, however, are that the doses were enormously high and the effect was specific to the rat.

Safety studies are done with a control group (vehicle only) and exposure to low doses (one- to four-fold multiples of efficacious dose), mid-doses (to determine dose–responsiveness) and high doses (to identify organ toxicity). Hopefully these types of studies will give an understanding of the range between efficacy and toxicity, the maximum achievable dose, the kinetics of achieving those doses and an idea of the anticipated toxicity. Endpoints for such studies are body weight and food consumption, ophthalmological effects, electrocardiography, clinical observations, mortality, organ weights and hepatic cytochrome P450 analyses. Also, macroscopic and microscopic examination of tissue is done; this can be extensive as thousands of tissue samples are analyzed (in addition to thousands of samples for clinical pathology, hematology, blood coagulation, clinical chemistry and urinalysis). There are several schemes for conducting such repeat dosing experiments; two common ones are shown in

Fig. 10.2. As safety testing progresses, there is increasing rigor with respect to how data is collected, how much data is collected and how it is analyzed. Figure 10.3 shows a progression to GLP studies (good laboratory practice) where particular attention is paid to accurate documentation of effects, calibration and maintenance of instruments used in the studies (with attention to application of internal and external audit of procedures), and validation of relevant technology with the aim of reporting data in a regulated environment. Some studies conducted at this stage are given in Table 10.2.

Overall, traditional pharmacology predicts only 10% to 70% of all human adverse effects. In a study of 150 drugs, when only rodents were used 40% of human toxic events were observed, in contrast to 60% when a non-rodent species was used; when both a rodent and non-rodent species were included, the maximal detection of toxic effects were observed (up to 70%).[6] In spite of best efforts to detect adverse effects, if late stage toxicity is observed that has been missed in early safety testing, the question arises "why did this occur?" and "how can we be assured that it will not occur with the next

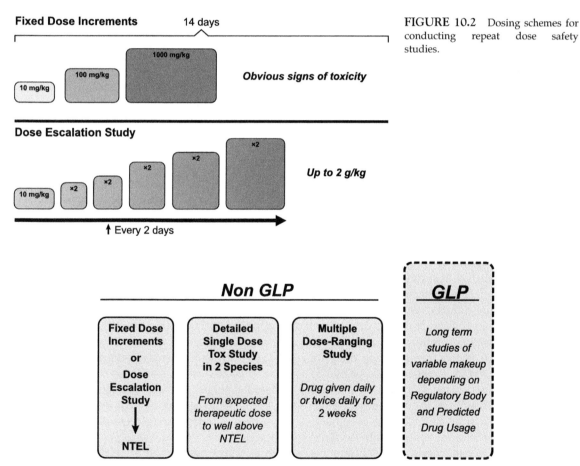

FIGURE 10.2 Dosing schemes for conducting repeat dose safety studies.

FIGURE 10.3 Repeat Dose Testing for observance of NOEL, NAOEL (also referred to as NTEL for no toxic effect levels). Once this has been done and progress is indicated, then GLP studies can be initiated.

TABLE 10.2   Types of Toxicity Tested for in GLP and Non-GLP Studies

Exploratory (Non-GLP) Studies

- *In vitro* screens
- *In silico* screens
- Cytotoxicity
- Immunotoxicity

- Hepatotoxicity
- Embryotoxicity
- Single and repeat dose range finding studies in two species

Regulatory (GLP) Studies

- Safety pharmacology
- Genotoxicity

- 24 months carcinogenicity in two species
- Reproductive toxicity in one species covering:
  - Fertility implantation
  - Fetal development
  - Pre/post natal effects

- 28-day repeat dose toxicity and recovery in two species
- 3–12 months' chronic toxicity in two species

candidate?" The basis of the answers to these questions lies in some of the basic assumptions made in safety testing. First, it is assumed that animal toxicity will translate to human toxicity and this encompasses assumptions about similar metabolites being formed and similar pharmacokinetics and sensitivity of organs to hazards. One prevalent problem is that animals are bred for health while drugs are usually targeted toward unhealthy individuals. This has led to proposals that more safety testing should be done in animal models of disease (i.e., rat models of type II diabetes, heterozygous p53 knockout mice for chemically induced carcinogenicity, lipopolysaccharide-induced inflammation (*vide infra*) and heterozygous superoxide dismutase-knockout mice to unveil mitochondrial toxicity). Another problem is that animals are bred for homogeneity to yield consistent experimental results, while the human population is much more diverse (60% of human genes may be alternatively spliced). In addition to the previously discussed case of bladder cancer with saccharin occurring only in rats, many other differences between animals and humans have been noted, such as increased liver weight to ketotifen only in dogs but not humans and renal necrosis to

efavirenz in rats but not humans. For these reasons there are proposals to utilize human tissue to a greater extent in safety testing in an effort to obviate differences due to species. Thus, human blood vessel endothelial cells,[7] hepatocytes[8] and human kidney proximal cells[9] have been used in safety studies for drug testing.

Another important difference is in the relative exposure to populations of varying size. Specifically, even in the most rigorous safety testing studies, the number of animals exposed to a drug is very much smaller than the numbers of humans that will be exposed to the drug as it becomes widely available to the greater human population (perhaps 1000–2000 animals exposed as opposed to 1,000,000 humans). Also, the dosage regimen given to animals in safety studies is tightly controlled whereas in the human population, dosages may sometimes be capricious (missed dosage, multiple dosages at one time, etc.). For example, Fig. 10.4 shows the increasing exposures of a drug to different populations as it progresses through development. For a drug such as Vioxx, which had a toxic event of one in every 113,927 patients, no clinical trial could have been devised to detect such an event (an incidence of 0.0009%). This also raises the

Toxicity through Stochastic Opportunity

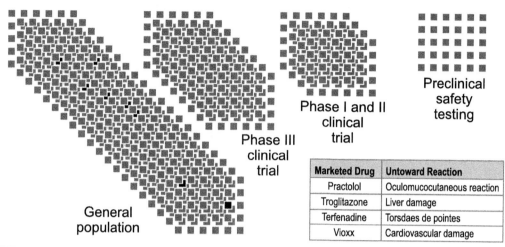

Marketed Drug	Untoward Reaction
Practolol	Oculomucocutaneous reaction
Troglitazone	Liver damage
Terfenadine	Torsdaes de pointes
Vioxx	Cardiovascular damage

FIGURE 10.4   Schematic diagram of increasing population exposure to a drug as it moves from discovery to development, and eventually to the marketplace in the general population. Shown in the box are four drugs found to produce serious toxic effects only when released to the greater population (see also Box 10.2).

question of the type of toxic effect involved, specifically if it depends on concentration (where exceeding a therapeutic window will always lead to toxicity) versus a toxicity due to stochastic opportunity. This latter classification of toxic effect (known as idiosyncratic) depends more on when a combination of rare conditions are encountered. It can be dependent on population, in that some populations may never show the effect. For these types of drugs various probabilities must be considered including the probability of exposure to drug, environmental risk factors and host risk factors (i.e., genetic predisposition to effect). These topics will be discussed further with mutagenicity and cancer, and idiosyncratic liver toxicity.

EARLY SAFETY TESTS

Just as with pharmacokinetics, there are avenues of exploration to assess safety that can be initiated very early on in the discovery and development process. For example, *in silico*

analysis of chemical structure can give guidance to chemists in terms of the identification of known substructures (toxicophores) that are present in known toxic compounds; these can be avoided in the optimization of primary and ADME activity. Figure 10.5 shows a number of common toxicophores present in known mutagenic compounds.

In addition to *in silico* studies there are some simple and inexpensive *in vitro* tests that can be done to assess possible harmful activity in molecules. These are:

1. **Interaction with receptors mediating autonomic function**: There are hundreds of extracellular receptors present on cell membranes that control the autonomic nervous system (sympathetic and parasympathetic control of cardiovascular, endocrine, gastrointestinal and central nervous system functions). Inappropriate activation of some of these by a drug intended for some other use can be detrimental; therefore candidate molecules

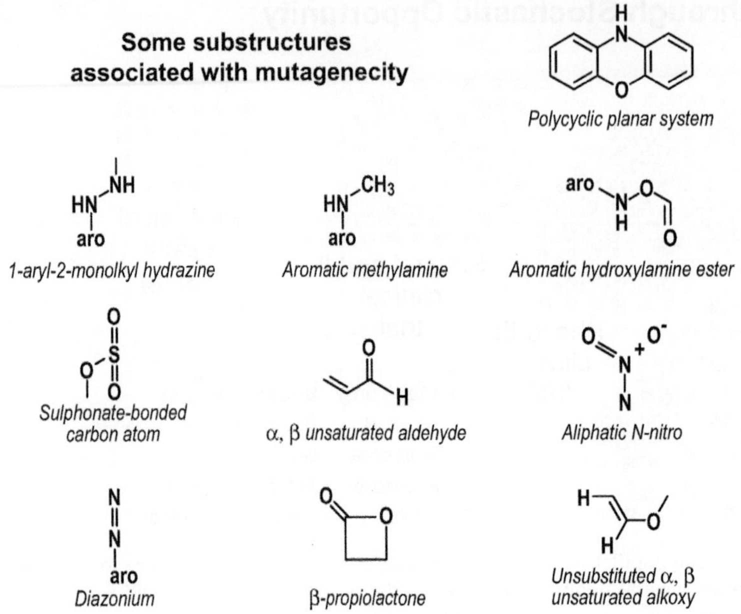

**Some substructures
associated with mutagenecity**

Polycyclic planar system

FIGURE 10.5 Some known toxico-phores identified as being common to mutagenic compounds (data from [12]).

1-aryl-2-monolkyl hydrazine

Aromatic methylamine

Aromatic hydroxylamine ester

Sulphonate-bonded carbon atom

α, β unsaturated aldehyde

Aliphatic N-nitro

Diazonium

β-propiolactone

Unsubstituted α, β unsaturated alkoxy

must be screened for any autonomic receptor activity. For example, activation of α-adrenoceptors (vasoconstriction leading to hypertension), β-adrenoceptors (tachycardia), antagonism of these (hypotension, cardiac failure) can lead to immediate and serious effects. While these effects are important, they are not difficult to detect in assays aimed at *in vitro* receptor function (and subsequent *in vivo* cardiovascular and behavioral studies). A list of common autonomic receptors that are routinely tested is given in Table 10.3.

2. **Blockade of hERG potassium channels**: This is an extremely serious effect whereby the ST segment in the human electrocardiogram is prolonged to the point where the critical communication between pacemaker cells in the atrium and the ventricle fails. This leads to a catastrophic cardiac event called *"Torsades de pointe"* which can cause syncope and sudden death.

The biological target mediating this event is the Human Ether-à-go-go Related Gene coding for the $K_V11.1$ potassium channel in the heart. This protein controls a repolarizing potassium current in the myocardium essential for the conduction of electrical current across the membrane to facilitate synchronous heartbeat. So important is this potential hazard, a number of approved drugs have been taken off the market when hERG activity was discovered (Fig. 10.6). There are simple binding or *in vitro* electrophysiological assays available to detect hERG activity which can be done early on in the development process. Definitive identification of QT prolongation is routinely explored through examination of EKG *in vivo*. There are documented cases where medicinal chemists have retained primary activity but eliminated this serious side-effect through structural changes in molecules.

TABLE 10.3 Some Common Autonomic Receptors for Unwanted Side-Effects

General Toxicity	GI Tract Toxicity	Cardiovascular Toxicity
5-HT_{2A}	5-HT_{1A}	5-HT_4
5-HT_{2B}	5-HT_{1P}	α_{1A}-adrenoceptor
α_{1A}-adrenoceptor	5-HT_{2A}	α_{1B}-adrenoceptor
α_{1B}-adrenoceptor	5-HT_{2B}	α_{2A}-adrenoceptor
α_{2A}-adrenoceptor	5-HT_3	α_{2B}-adrenoceptor
Adenosine 2A	5-HT_4	α_{2C}-adrenoceptor
Adenosine A1	α_{2A}-adrenoceptor	Adenosine 2A
β_1-adrenoceptor	α_{2B}-adrenoceptor	Adenosine A1
β_2-adrenoceptor	α_{2C}-adrenoceptor	Adenosine A3
Bradykinin B2	CCK2	Angiotensin AT1
Cannabinoid CB1	Dopamine D2	β_1-adrenoceptor
Dopamine D2	δ-opioid	β_2-adrenoceptor
Histamine H1	EP2	Bradykinin B1
μ opioid	EP3	Bradykinin B2
Muscarinic m1	Gastrin	Cannabinoid CB1
Purinergic P2Y1	Histamine H2	CGRP
	μ opioid	Dopamine D2
	Motilin	Endothelin A
	Muscarinic m2	Endothelin B
	Muscarinic m3	Histamine H3
	SST1	Muscarinic m1
	VIP	Muscarinic m2
		Muscarinic m3
		Muscarinic m4
		Nicotinic Ach
		NPY_1
		Thromboxane A2
		Vasopressin V_{1a}
		Vasopressin V_{1b}

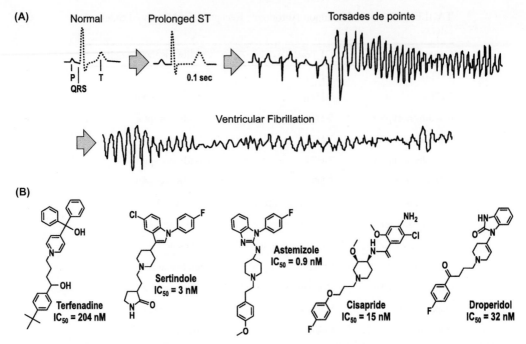

FIGURE 10.6 (A) Blockade of the hERG potassium channel in the heart leads to QT segment prolongation in the electrocardiogram and subsequent arrhythmia and ventricular fibrillation (*Torsades de pointe*). (B) Five drugs with nanomolar potency for this effect that have been withdrawn from the market.

3. **Cytotoxicity**: This refers to any effect that eventually could lead to cell death (cyto from the Greek *kytos* meaning hollow and toxic from the Greek *toxikon* meaning arrow poison). Cells are extremely complex bodies with a temporally diverse lifetime (i.e., different processes are important to life at different times); therefore defining drug effects that will interfere with these process can be speculative if no clear lethal effect is seen. A commonly used simple assay is the MTT cell proliferation assay (see Fig. 10.7). The basis for this assay is the fact that mitochondrial function is essential to cell health; addition of the substrate for mitochondrial reductase MTT (3-(4,5-dimethylthiazol-2-yl)-2,5-diphenyltetrazolium bromide), which is colored yellow, leads to the formation of formazan in healthy mitochondria (colored purple). This furnishes a simple colorimetric assay for cell health where comparison of the color of cell cultures (one control and one drug treated) leads to estimates of the number of living cells. It should be noted that drugs that affect metabolic function can give conflicting signals in the MTT test. There are numerous other ways to show cellular toxicity, from cessation of growth to losing membrane integrity (and subsequent production of necrosis). Membrane integrity can be measured with trypan blue or propidium iodide substances that are normally excluded from healthy cells. Cells can also activate a genetic program of cell death (apoptosis) which produces distinctive markers. In general, cell nuclear morphology, mitochondrial function,

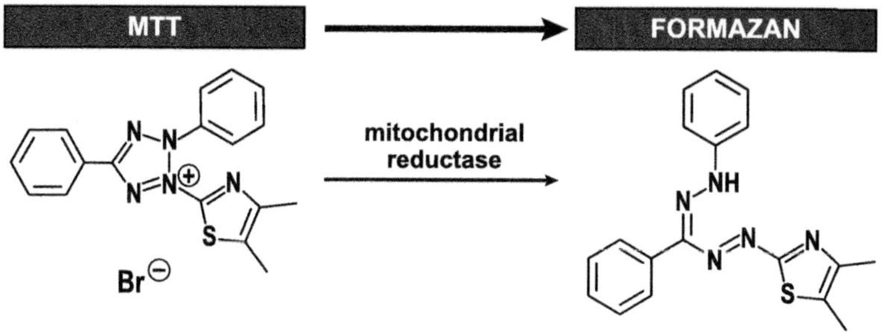

FIGURE 10.7 MTT cell proliferation assay for cytotoxicity. Mitochondrial function is assessed through the level of activity of mitochondrial reductase converting the yellow substrate MTT (3-(4,5-dimethylthiazol-2-yl)-2,5-diphenyltetrazolium bromide) to the purple product formazan. Colorimetric comparison of control cells and cells exposed to a test compound in varying concentrations can yield a dose−response curve for remaining living cells in culture.

plasma membrane integrity and speed of proliferation can all be used to measure cell health, and all of these effects can be readily obtained from *in vitro* assays in cell culture.

4. **Mutagenicity**: The ability of a drug to induce mutation in a cell can be indicative of possible carcinogenic activity. A simple and rapid test for drug mutagenicity is the Ames test. Developed by Bruce Ames and his group at the University of California Berkely, this tests the ability of a molecule to produce changes in the DNA of a modified *Salmonella tryphimurium* (a bacteria modified to maximize the probability of mutation). Specifically, unlike native bacteria, the Ames bacterium is engineered such that it cannot synthesize histidine (and therefore requires it in the medium to live and grow). If no mutation occurs, the culture containing the Ames bacteria will die. However, if mutation occurs, it often confers the capability to synthesize histidine (and thus live in histidine free media) upon the organism. Therefore, if cells grow in histidine free media, it is likely that mutation has occurred (see Fig. 10.8). The bacterium and media are altered in other ways to maximize the probability of mutation. Specifically, the lipopolysaccharide coat of the bacterium is compromised to allow maximal entry of

compounds and the DNA repair capability of the bacterium is reduced. In addition, S9 hepatic enzyme fraction (see Chapter 7) is added to the medium to maximize the probability of formation of metabolites that would be seen *in vivo* with the compound. This is a rapid and extremely useful test but as with all tests of stochastic probability it is not always predictive (see Box 10.3).

HEPATIC TOXICITY

As discussed in Chapters 7 and 8, the liver is the primary organ of detoxification for the body. Moreover, the liver receives the highest initial dose of all drugs given orally due to the first pass effect. Therefore, it perhaps should not be surprising that drug-induced liver injury is the most frequent cause of withdrawal of approved drugs; this organ is on the front line for the detection of toxic effects. There are two general types of drug-induced liver injury: intrinsic hepatotoxicity (occurs in all individuals in a dose-dependent, and thus predictable, manner) and idiosyncratic hepatotoxicity (results from a succession of unlikely events). This latter type of hepatotoxicity is much more difficult to detect since it depends on the frequency of reaction in animal studies invariably involving small numbers. In

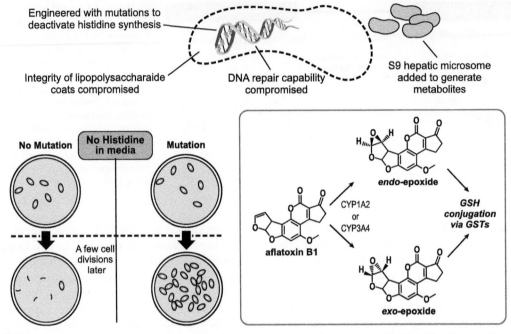

FIGURE 10.8 The Ames test. Engineered *Salmonella typhimurium* (which cannot grow in hisitidine-free medium unless a mutation has occurred) is cultured in hisitidine-free medium. If compound is added and the culture grows, it is likely that a mutation has been induced by the compound. Inset shows an example of a mutagenic product formed from aflatoxin by the hepatic enzyme CYP3A4.

BOX 10.3

THE PROBLEM OF PREDICTING MUTAGENICITY

Dioxin (common name for 2,3,7,8-tetrachloro-dibenzo-p-dioxin) is an extremely toxic substance that, when ingested, can lead to enzyme induction, immunotoxicity, reproductive and endocrine effects, developmental toxicity, chloracne and tumor promotion. In spite of its clearly documented mutagenic activity, dioxin is not positive in the Ames test.[14] Nitroglycerin (commonly used for the treatment of angina), on the other hand, is mutagenic in the Ames test. These data highlight the stochastic nature of mutagenicity and the difficulty of predicting it.

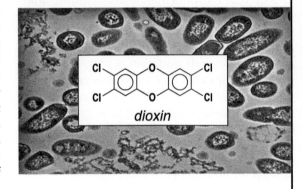

TABLE 10.4 Comparison of Intrinsic and Idiosynchratic Hepatoxicity

Intrinsic	Idiosynchratic
• Affects all individuals at some dose	• Attacks only susceptible individuals
• Clearly dose-related	• Unclear relation to dose
• Predictable latent period after exposure	• Variable onset relative to exposure
• Predictable with routine animal testing	• Not predictable with routine animal testing
	• Variable liver pathology

addition, interspecies variation and genetic variability play a significant role in these effects (there 1.4 million single nucleotide polymorphisms in the human genome and 78 polymorphisms of the hepatic enzyme CYP2D6 alone). Some features of intrinsic and idiosyncratic hepatotoxicity are compared in Table 10.4.

It is difficult to deal with idiosyncratic hepatotoxicity; for example the drug for arthritis diclofenac produces serious hepatotoxicity in 6 of every 100,000 patients (8–20% of those develop diclofenac jaundice and die of liver failure). Such extremely low incidence (0.006%) makes it difficult to detect and difficult to predict in new drug testing. Thus, only one half of new drugs that produce hepatotoxicity in clinical stages of development show *any* animal toxicity. One hypothesis put forward to explain some of the capriciousness surrounding idiosyncratic hepatotoxicity is that, in these cases, the threshold for observing intrinsic hepatotoxicity is greater than the lethal dose (thus it is never routinely observed). However, genetic, environmental, stress (i.e., arthritis, viral hepatitis, bacterial infection, periodontal disease, asthma) and other factors may shift the threshold for this intrinsic hepatotoxicity to much lower levels periodically and when this occurs idiosyncratic hepatotoxicity appears (see

Fig. 10.9). One experimental approach to predict this is to chemically stress the liver to mimic these threshold lowering effects; this can be done with non-toxic doses of gram-negative bacterial source lipopolysaccharide (LPS).[10] This procedure has been shown to sensitize the liver to the toxic effects of carbon tetrachloride, monocrotaline, cocaine, aflatoxin B1, diclofenax and sulindac. In addition, there are a number of physiologically based biochemical assays that can be used to assess liver function (and liver damage) including the appearance of steatosis (accumulation of fatty acids), intrahepatic cholestasis (impairment of bile formation), liver microsomal glutathione levels (to test for reactive intermediates) and assays of phospholipidosis (accumulation of phospholipids).

SUMMARY

- The main aim of safety pharmacology is to define the optimal way in which potentially valuable drugs can be utilized without causing harm.
- An important difference between testing for primary activity and ADME properties and safety is that, in the former, what to look for is defined; in safety testing it is not known what should be looked for. Under these circumstances, a great many tests must be undertaken to develop confidence that harmful effects will not be seen.
- There are generally two types of toxicity; intrinsic toxicity which is related to drug exposure (if enough drug is administered, the effect will appear) and that due to stochastic opportunity (idiosyncratic).This latter event is rare and difficult to predict.
- Even with exhaustive testing, once a drug enters the greater population, very rare negative events (the probability of which may be infintesmal in drug development testing) may be found.

(A)

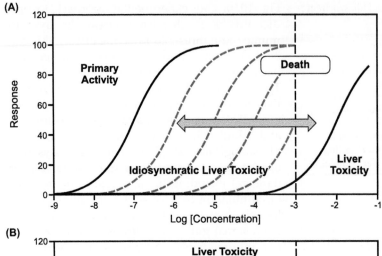

(B)

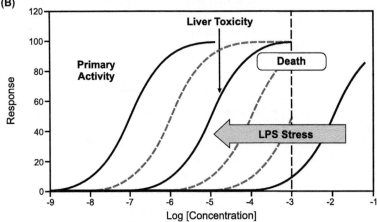

FIGURE 10.9 Idiosyncratic hepatotoxicity. (A) Extremely rare hepatotoxic events may be so because, for a given compound, the intrinsic hepatotoxicity threshold in a normal liver may lie above the lethal dose (and thus may never be seen). However, conditions of stress may move this threshold to much lower levels to unveil hepatotoxicity which may then appear random. Experimental procedures such as LPS stress (see text) may reduce the threshold for liver toxicity and thus uncover what would be seen as rare idiosyncratic hepatotoxicity in a larger population (drawn from [10]).

- There are some common simple *in vitro* tests to quickly detect chemical scaffolds that interact with autonomic receptors, block the hERG channel, are cytotoxic and may be mutagenic. These can be carried out early in the development process.
- Hepatotoxicity is a very common toxic drug effect due to the fact that high concentrations of drugs reach the liver. Moreover, the liver is designed to chemically interact with drugs. Sensitization of liver assays to toxic effects may assist in detection of rare idiosyncratic hepatotoxicity.

QUESTIONS

10.1 What are two general types of toxicity and which one is most difficult to deal with?

10.2 A promising new antihypertensive was progressed to *in vivo* safety studies and no toxic effects were noted. This is both a good and bad thing; why?

10.3 A series of compounds was subjected to Ames testing and found not to cause mutation. Should the conclusion be that these compounds are not mutagenic and thus would not cause cancer?

10.4 An optimistic and a pessimistic biologist were both members of a discovery team that delivered a new drug that passed Phase II testing and was destined for final Phase III testing. Most of the safety studies were complete and a large safety margin appeared to be operative for the compound. The optimist declared "we made it" while the pessimist countered with "not yet." What is the basis for the pessimist's point of view?

References

[1] R. Eri, J.R. Jonsson, N. Pandeya, D.M. Purdie, A.D. Clouston, N. Martin, et al., CCR5-Delta32 mutation is strongly associated with primary sclerosing cholangitis, Genes Immun. 5 (2004) 444–450.

[2] W.G. Glass, D.H. McDermott, J.K. Lim, S. Lekhong, S.F. Yu, J. Pape, et al., CCR5 deficiency increases risk of symptomatic Nile virus infection, J. Exp. Med. 203 (2006) 35–40.

[3] C. Moench, A. Uhrig, A.W. Lohse, G. Otto, CC chemokine receptor 5delta32 polymorphism – a risk factor for ischemic-type biliary lesions following orthotopic liver transplantation, Liver Transpl. 10 (2004) 434–439.

[4] E. De Silva, M.P. Stumpf, HIV and CCR5-Δ32 resistance allele, FEMS Microbiol. Lett. 241 (2004) 1–12.

[5] P. Greaves, A. Williams, M. Eve, First dose of potential new medicines to humans: How animals help, Nature Rev. Drug. Disc. 3 (2003) 226–236.

[6] R. Dixit, U.A. Boelsteri, Healthy animals and models of human diseases in safety assessment of human pharmaceuticals, including therapeutic antibodies, Drug Disc. Today 12 (2007) 236–342.

[7] C. Schleger, S.J. Platz, U. Deschl, Development of an in vitro model for vascular injury with human endothelial cells, Altex 21(Suppl. 3) (2004) 12–19.

[8] J.T. MacGregor, J.M. Collins, Y. Sugiyama, C.A. Tyson, J. Dean, L. Smith, et al., In vitro human tissue models in risk assessment: Report of a consensus-building workshop, Toxicol. Sci. 59 (2001) 17–36.

[9] W. Li, D.F. Choy, M.S. Lam, T. Morgan, M.E. Sullivan, J.M. Post, Use of cultured cells of kidney origin to assess specific cytotoxic effects of nephrotoxins, Toxicol. In Vitro 17 (2003) 107–113.

[10] R.A. Roth, P.E. Ganey, Intrinsic versus idiosyncratic drug-induced hepatotoxicity: Two villains or one? J. Pharmacol. Exp. Ther. 332 (2010) 692–697.

[11] M.N. Cayen, Prediction of pharmacokinetics and drug safety in humans, in: P.L. Bullock (Ed.), Early Drug Development, John Wiley and Sons, New York, 2010, pp. 89–129.

[12] J. Kazius, R. McGuire, R. Bursi, Derivation and validation of toxicophores for mutagenicity prediction, J. Med. Chem. 48 (2005) 312–320.

[13] B.K. Park, M. Pirmohamed, N.R. Kitteringham, Idiosyncratic drug reactions: A mechanistic evaluation of risk, Br. J. Clin. Pharmacol. 34 (1992) 377–395.

[14] L.E. Geiger, R.A. Neal, Mutagenicity testing of 2,3,7,8-tetrachlorodibenzo-p-dioxin in histidine auxotrophs of Salmonella typhimurium, Toxicol. Applied Pharmacol. 59 (1981) 125–129.

Appendix A: Answers to Chapter Questions

CHAPTER 1

1.1 What is the main value of the receptor concept in pharmacology and physiology?

By defining a common point of origin for the action of a hormone or other endogenous transmitter in the body, receptors insert order into an otherwise diverse collection of physiological responses. This order promotes pharmacological intervention since it gives a point where chemicals can modify these processes.

1.2 How is potency characterized in a dose–response curve?

The potency is the concentration of drug that gives a defined response. For example, in an *in vitro* experiment the pEC_{50} is the negative logarithm of the molar concentration of an agonist that produces 50% of the maximal response to the agonist. Thus, a $pEC_{50} = 8.3$ means that 50% of the maximal response to the agonist is produced by a concentration of 5 nM.

1.3 Define full agonist, partial agonist, antagonist, inverse agonist.

A full agonist produces a drug-mediated maximal response that is equal to the maximal response that the system can produce; a partial agonist produces a drug maximal response that is lower than the maximal response that the system can produce. An antagonist produces no overt response but does inhibit the response to an agonist that normally does produce a response. An inverse agonist reverses the basal response of the system when it is due to spontaneous receptor activation (constitutive activity).

1.4 Why can the potency of an agonist change when it is tested in different tissues?

The actual potency of an agonist depends upon two drug-related parameters (affinity and efficacy) and two tissue related parameters (target density and efficiency of stimulus-response coupling). These latter two factors can vary greatly in different tissues. Thus, the ways in which drug targets are coupled to cellular response mechanisms and the actual number of targets themselves can cause variation in agonist potency as agonists are tested in different cell types.

1.5 Upon what major assumption is the null method for comparing agonist potency based?

The major assumption in this procedure is that both drugs produce cellular response via the same mechanism. This can be an issue for agonists of receptors that bias the stimulus to various pathways in a multi-pathway cellular system. When potency ratios are used to compare the relative activity of agonists in different systems, it is assumed that the stimulus-response machinery in the system is monotonic, i.e., there is one value of y for every value of x.

CHAPTER 2

2.1 The response to a test agonist is not blocked by conventional antagonists of the target but does not appear in a recombinant system where the target is not present in the cell. What could be happening?

The agonist may activate the target allosterically by binding to a site that is not blocked by the antagonist. However, the agonist specifically activates the target to produce a response; therefore in a recombinant cell line where the target is not present, the agonist cannot produce an effect.

2.2 Drug A has an equilibrium dissociation constant (K_{eq}) of 10^{-8} M while drug B has a K_{eq} of 10^{-10} M. Which drug has the higher affinity and why?

The K_{eq} is the molar concentration of molecule that binds to 50% of the surface or binding sites. Drug B has the higher affinity since it takes a much lower concentration of Drug B (than Drug A) to bind 50% of the sites

2.3 Two agonists produce a response in a system both with a pEC_{50} of 7.5. However, one produces 25% maximal response while the other produces 90% maximal response. What is the difference between these two agonists?

The two agonists differ in efficacy. The higher efficacy agonist produces 90% maximal response while the lower efficacy agonist produces only 25% maximal response.

2.4 The potency ratio for two full agonists A and B is 15.4 in one cellular system and 2.3 in another. What does this lack of correlation of full agonist potency ratio suggest?

If the molecular mechanism of agonism for two full agonists is identical, then cellular potency ratios in any cell type will be constant. However, if they produce agonism through activation of different cellular mechanisms (i.e., stabilize different active conformation states of the target protein) then variation in whole cell potency ratios can result. These

data suggest that agonists A and B produce agonism through stabilization of different target active states

CHAPTER 3

3.1 Why did Black and Leff use the Michaelis—Menten equation as the basis for signal transduction in the operational model?

The shape of the relationship between agonist concentration and cellular response is very similar to the relationship between substrate concentration and enzyme velocity as defined by the Michaelis—Menten model.

3.2 Describe how the operational model parameter τ characterizes both the intrinsic efficacy of the agonist and the sensitivity of the system.

The parameter τ is the ratio of the receptor density $[R_t]$ and K_E, the equilibrium dissociation constant of the agonist-bound receptor interaction with the cellular signaling components. Low values of K_E signify an efficient coupling of the receptor to cellular response mechanisms and also that the [AR] complex is a highly effective instigator of response (i.e., that agonist A has high intrinsic efficacy). Thus the sensitivity of the system is characterized by $[R_t]$ and an element of K_E, and the intrinsic efficacy of the agonist by another element of K_E.

3.3 A given agonist A was found to have a receptor reserve of 90% in a given tissue system. What does this mean? Another agonist B had a reserve in the same tissue of only 40%; what properties of agonists A and B could lead to this result?

A receptor reserve of 90% means that only 10% of the available receptors need to be activated by agonist A to produce the tissue maximal response. The fact that agonist B had a reserve of 40% means that it requires 60% of the receptor population to produce the same (maximal) response. This indicates that agonist B has a lower efficacy than agonist A.

CHAPTER 4

4.1 A given orthosteric antagonist produces a shift to the right of the agonist dose–response curve with no depression of maximum and a further shift with a depression of maximum at higher doses. What might be happening?

The antagonist may be a pseudo-irreversible slow offset antagonist producing non-competitive blockade of the agonist. This could be a system of high receptor reserve for the agonist (i.e., only a fraction of the receptor population need be activated to achieve maximal response); therefore low levels of irreversible blockade of receptors produce a shift but no depression of maximum. Higher levels of receptor blockade, beyond the receptor reserve for the agonist, then produce a depressed maximum to the agonist.

4.2 A rapid estimate of the potency of an antagonist of unknown potency is required. What would be a good method of doing this?

The blockade of a steady-state 80% of maximal agonist response with a range of concentrations of the test antagonist would yield a pIC_{50} to rapidly estimate antagonist potency.

4.3 A given antagonist produces surmountable simple competitive blockade in one type of assay and a depression of agonist maximal response in another. The chemist is worried that there is a problem in the testing; why should this not be a concern?

Surmountable versus insurmountable orthosteric antagonism is a kinetic condition which can result from differences in the time allowed in an assay to visualize agonist response. Thus, slow offset antagonists can produce surmountable blockade in assays allowing long periods to collect responses and insurmountable antagonism in assays where this window is small.

4.4 A pIC_{50} is measured for an antagonist and surprisingly, the maximal response for antagonism falls well below the basal response of the assay. What could be happening and what does this say about the antagonist in question?

This suggests that the system has constitutive activity (i.e., the basal response is an elevated response due to spontaneous activation of receptors) and that the antagonist is an inverse agonist that reverses this elevated basal activity down to true zero (no activation) levels.

CHAPTER 5

5.1 A given antagonist was found to produce potent surmountable blockade with a pA_2 value of 8.0. When investigators used 100 times the pA_2 concentration (10^{-6}M) in an attempt to completely block a process, they were surprised to find that the process was still not blocked and partially operative (only a four-fold shift of the curve appeared). What could be happening?

This could very well be saturation of allosteric effect with a maximal effect of the allosteric antagonist of a 4-fold reduction in sensitivity (the allosteric ligand produces a maximal four-fold diminution of receptor function).

5.2 A discovery effort was aimed at potentiating insulin release through the GLP-1 receptor and accordingly, a screen was run to detect PAMs. To facilitate the mechanics of the screen, a stable analog of the natural agonist for the GLP-1 receptor, exendin, was used. Subsequent lead optimization of hits showed an alarming lack of correspondence of effect in a natural system of insulin release; why might this occur?

This could be probe dependence where the allosteric molecules detected by the assay with exendin have different allosteric effects on the physiological natural agonist *in vivo*.

5.3 A given antagonism is found to produce a 50% depression of the maximal response to an agonist at a concentration of 10 nM. What experiments can be done to determine if this effect is steric blockade (orthosteric antagonism) or allosteric modulation?

An orthosteric non-competitive antagonist, if given in sufficiently high concentration, will block the responsiveness of the system to baseline (maximal response to the agonist of zero). Therefore, the antagonist should be tested at a concentration of $1 \mu M$ (100-fold increase in concentration) to see if this occurs. Also, a range of other agonists should be tested to try to uncover probe dependence.

5.4 The pK_B of an allosteric antagonist for a chemokine receptor measured to be 8.2 for blocking the effects of the chemokine CCL5. However, as a blocker of CCL3 (a different chemokine) it was found to be 7.5. What could be causing this difference?

The values for α are different for the co-binding ligands CCL5 and CCL3. The observed affinity is an amalgam of pK_B, α and β values.

10 nM. In contrast, there was no significant antitumor activity found *in vivo*. What could be the issues and how could they be addressed?

The compound needs to be absorbed *in vivo* and have a sufficient half-life to be present in the extracellular medium to enter the tumor cell via bulk diffusion or active uptake. These barriers may be preventing the molecule from accessing the kinase *in vivo*. A first step would be test the molecule in an *in vitro* cell culture for kinase inhibition to confirm that it can enter the cell.

6.2 ATP levels in a cell can be high; therefore competitive inhibitors of kinases can have correspondingly low potency. What would be a good type of enzyme inhibitor for this type of scenario?

An uncompetitive inhibitor becomes more potent under conditions of high substrate availability. Under these conditions, an uncompetitive kinase inhibitor would be more active in cells if ATP levels are high.

6.3 The IC_{50} for a test enzyme inhibitor was found to be 30 nM when measured at 60 minutes and 25 nM at 120 minutes. In one assay, the IC_{50} was not measured until 600 minutes and was found to be 12 nM. Could this be indicative of a problem, and if so, why?

A reversible mass action driven association process that comes to near completion (30 nM to 25 nM) in 120 minutes should not change at 600 minutes unless it is a very slow onset irreversible inhibition. The compound could be irreversible showing mechanism-based and/or time-dependent enzyme inhibition.

CHAPTER 6

6.1 A biochemical kinase assay showed that a test compound for cancer had an IC_{50} of

CHAPTER 7

7.1 An active scaffold was found to be very insoluble in water. The team decided that this would "not be a problem" as an emulsion could be given that would be absorbed. Why are they wrong?

All drugs must dissolve in water before they can take part in any physiological process such as transfer across membranes.

7.2 A drug discovery team was asked if they needed ADME support early in their program and they declined stating "we can build in the ADME properties after we get the lead." Why are they wrong?

The structure activity relationships governing primary activity can be (and often are) completely different from those controlling ADME properties. It is very difficult to make a molecule ADME friendly if it is already optimized for another activity.

7.3 What are some *in vitro* assays available to estimate the stability of a molecule to hepatic degradation?

Microsomes (chopped liver centrifuged to enzyme containing membranes), S9 (a centrifuge fraction containing more types of enzymes than microsomes) or hepatocytes (isolated liver cells).

7.4 Why are discovery teams so worried about drug–drug interactions?

These can be serious and life-threatening. They are also expected as rarely is your new drug given to a patient who is not already on other drugs. These patients are titrated to doses of their drugs and a new drug could upset the balanced titration and lead to serious side-effects.

7.5 A drug candidate was tested in rats via the oral route after it was found to have a huge rate of permeation (38 cm s^{-1}) in the CaCo-2 *in vitro* permeation assay. The drug was not even detectable in rats indicating no bioavailability; what could be happening?

This candidate should have been tested in liver microsomes first as it is probably highly metabolized by the liver. To be bioavailable via the oral route, a drug must survive the "first pass effect" which is absorption followed by passage straight into the liver through the portal vein for hepatic metabolism.

7.6 An investigational drug is found to cause the effect of another drug being used to treat the patient to lose its effect. What is one mechanism that can cause this effect?

Liver induction. The investigational drug may cause induction of cytochrome P450 enzymes in the patient's liver to increase their levels and thus increase the metabolism of the other drug.

CHAPTER 8

8.1 What is clearance?

This is the process of the drug leaving the body (not redistributing within the body compartments). It is expressed as the rate of cleansing a given volume of body water completely of the drug per unit time.

8.2 A volume of distribution for a new drug was found to 159 liters. How could this be if a human normally has about 40 liters total body water?

The sample is taken from the central compartment (circulation) while the drug may be accumulating elsewhere in the body. This makes the central compartment concentration very low which, when calculated with the total amount of drug given to the patient, makes it appear that the drug is dissolved in a huge volume of water. Clinicians are sampling from a region where the drug is absent.

8.3 Clinicians are able to control seizures in a patient through careful monitoring of an intravenous drip. As the dosage increases, suddenly the concentration of drug in the patient rises sharply to overdose levels; what could be happening?

The increasing dosage may be saturating a steady-state process in the body to push the system into non-linear pharmacokinetics.

8.4 A drug is given as a single i.v. injection and the concentration monitored. The initial $t_{1/2}$ is 5 minutes, indicating a rapid elimination but this changes to a $t_{1/2}$ of 2 hours. What happened?

The initial $t_{1/2}$ reflects the drug distribution throughout the body through various compartments and does not reflect elimination. Once the drug has distributed, then the $t_{1/2}$ reflects true clearance (elimination) of the drug

8.5 A given investigational drug was extremely well absorbed via the oral route and had a $t_{1/2}$ of 9 hours (adequate for once-a-day dosing). Unfortunately, the safety margin for this compound was limited as toxic effects were seen at 2.5 times the C_{max} for the dose used. What is a strategy that could be employed to make this compound more reliable and therapeutically useful?

The potential hazard with a well absorbed but toxic drug is attainment of toxic C_{max} levels. Formulations to retard the rate of absorption (i.e., coated tablets) could reduce the likelihood of high C_{max} levels.

CHAPTER 9

9.1 An agonist for β-adrenoceptors has excellent permeation properties *in vivo* and a low value for clearance. In addition, this compound is extremely potent in cell culture cyclic AMP studies *in vitro* ($pEC_{50} = 8.1$). In spite of this profile, the *in vivo* profile is disappointing and little

bronchodilation was observed. What could be happening?

It should be determined if the high activity *in vitro* is due to high affinity or high efficacy. A high affinity but low efficacy agonist could be extremely potent in a sensitive system and have very low activity in a low sensitivity system.

9.2 An antitumor compound was active against xenograft tumors in mice but proved to be disappointing in humans. Analysis of total compound showed plasma levels to be comparable eliminating differences in pharmacokinetics to be the cause. What else could be occurring?

While total drug level can be measured from plasma samples, the amount of drug free to interact with tissue (i.e., not plasma protein bound) is the important factor in determining *in vivo* efficacy. It could be in this case that the drug is highly protein bound in humans but not mice.

9.3 Two anticholinergic antagonists of comparable potency *in vitro* are tested for hyperactive urinary bladder *in vivo*. One shows clearly superior effects over the other even though both have comparable levels of clearance and plasma protein binding. What additional experiments would be useful to examine this problem?

The kinetics of receptor dissociation should be tested for these antagonists to see if one has a slower rate of dissociation from the target (and thus gives better target coverage *in vivo*).

9.4 A β$_2$-adrenoceptor agonist for alleviation of airway constriction in asthma is found to be six-fold more potent in relaxing constricted airway muscle than in producing harmful tachycardia in experiments done *in vitro*. While this ratio is not considered high and suggests that the compound would have dangerous cardiovascular effects, it is still worth testing *in vivo*. Why?

If the agonist is given via aerosol, there will be a concentration gradient from the airways (highest) to the general circulation (lower) therefore the concentrations reaching the heart will be considerably lower than those activating the airways. Also, plasma protein binding and clearance pharmacokinetics may further give a favorable gradient between the airways and the heart. *In vivo* effects may provide a further margin of safety for this agonist so it should be tested *in vivo*.

CHAPTER 10

10.1 What are two general types of toxicity and which one is most difficult to deal with?

Intrinsic toxicity (concentration dependent) is straightforward to deal with as it occurs at all times a given threshold of drug level is exceeded. Idiosyncratic toxicity occurs as a result of stochastic probability and can depend on a variety of other probabilities. This is difficult to predict and may be exceedingly rare though serious.

10.2 A promising new antihypertensive was progressed to *in vivo* safety studies and no toxic effects were noted. This is both a good and bad thing; why?

This is a good observation from the point of view that the compound appears safe (providing therapeutic falls in blood pressure were seen). However, drug exposure must continue until some untoward effects are seen in order to define the safety margin for the drug; some bad things must be seen to quantify the safety ratio for the good things.

10.3 A series of compounds was subjected to Ames testing and found not to cause mutation. Should the conclusion be that these compounds are not mutagenic and thus would not cause cancer?

Results from the Ames test must be put in the perspective that this test does not necessarily detect **all** carcinogenic and mutagenic compounds and, also, even if a compound is mutagenic, it still may not be carcinogenic. However, on balance, a negative result in the Ames test (no mutation) is generally good but carcinogenicity can still occur in further testing, whereas a positive result in the Ames test is a harbinger that the compound will be mutagenic and possibly carcinogenic.

10.4 An optimistic and a pessimistic biologist were both members of a discovery team that delivered a new drug that passed Phase II testing and was destined for final Phase III testing. Most of the safety studies were complete and a large safety margin appeared to be operative for the compound. The optimist declared "we made it" while the pessimist countered with "not yet." What is the basis for the pessimist's point of view?

The compound has not yet seen a large enough population of subjects to detect rare but serious idiosyncratic toxic effects. Confidence builds as the Phase III trials are completed but there are cases of drugs that show serious idiosyncratic effects beyond Phase III (Box 10.2).

Appendix B: Derivations and Proofs

B1 SUCCESSIVE SATURABLE FUNCTIONS LEADS TO AMPLIFICATION OF SIGNALS

For Chapter 1

In a cell, biochemical reactions function in series whereby the product of one reaction becomes the substrate for the next, etc. In these types of systems, the sensitivity of the complete system to an initial substrate will always be higher than the sensitivity of any one step in the system. Thus, the K_{eq} for a series of reactions will always be of lower magnitude than the K_{eq} for any one step.

Cellular stimulus–response coupling is represented by a series arrangement of saturable functions of the form:

$$Output_1 = \frac{[input_1]}{[input_1] + K_1} \qquad (B.1)$$

Under these circumstances, the midpoint (sensitivity) of the function defined by equation B.1 is K_1. A series arrangement leads to the output from one function becoming the input for the next, thus the output from a second function in the series is:

$$Output_2 = \frac{[Output_1]}{[Output_1] + K_2} \qquad (B.2)$$

Substituting for $output_1$ from equation B.1, the equation for $output_2$ is:

$$Output_2 = \frac{[input_1]}{[input_1](1 + K_2) + K_1 K_2} \qquad (B.3)$$

Rearranging to isolate $input_1$ yields:

$$Output_2 = \frac{[input_1]}{[input_1] + \frac{K_1 K_2}{(1 + K_2)}} \qquad (B.4)$$

The sensitivity for $output_2$ (denoted $K_{observed}$), in terms of $input_1$, is given by:

$$K_{observed} = \frac{K_1 K_2}{(1 + K_2)} \qquad (B.5)$$

It can be seen from equation B.5 that for all non-zero values of K_2, $(1 + K_2) > K_2$, $K_{observed}$ will always be $< K_1$. Thus, the equilibrium constant for the series of reactions is always less than the equilbrium constant for a single reaction. This means that series saturable functions always amplify initial signals.

B2 THE POTENCY OF A FULL AGONIST DEPENDS ON BOTH AFFINITY AND EFFICACY

For Chapter 2

Denoting the affinity of a molecule as K_A and the efficacy as τ (see Chapter 3 for details on this parameter), the response to an agonist is given by (see Chapter 3 for explanation of this equation and B.3 for derivation):

$$\text{Response} = \frac{E_m \bullet [A] \bullet \tau}{[A](1 + \tau) + K_A} \quad (B.6)$$

where E_m is the maximal response of the system. It can be seen that as $[A] \to \infty$, the maximal response (Max) is given by:

$$\text{Max} = \frac{E_m \bullet \tau}{(1 + \tau)} \quad (B.7)$$

Defining the EC_{50} as the point where response is half maximal E_m defines the following equality:

$$0.5 = \frac{[EC_{50}](1 + \tau)}{[EC_{50}](1 + \tau) + K_A} \quad (B.8)$$

Under these circumstances, the equation for EC_{50} for a partial agonist reduces to:

$$EC_{50} = \frac{K_A}{(1 + \tau)} \quad (B.9)$$

It can be seen from B.9 that EC_{50} is a function of both affinity (K_A) and efficacy (τ).

B3 DERIVATION OF THE BLACK–LEFF OPERATIONAL MODEL

For Chapter 3

Beginning with a form of the Michaelis–Menten equation for enzymes:

$$\text{Response} = \frac{[A]E_m}{[A] + \nu} \quad (B.10)$$

where the concentration of agonist is $[A]$, E_m is the maximal response of the system and ν is a fitting parameter for the hyperbolic function, the concentration of drug $[A]$ can be expressed as:

$$[A] = \frac{\text{Response} \bullet \nu}{E_m[A] - \text{Response}} \quad (B.11)$$

Mass action defines the concentration of agonist–receptor complex as:

$$[AR] = \frac{[A] \cdot [R_t]}{[A] + K_A} \quad (B.12)$$

where $[R_t]$ is the receptor density and K_A is the equilibrium dissociation constant of the agonist–receptor complex. A second function for $[A]$ can then be derived:

$$[A] = \frac{[AR] \cdot K_A}{[R_t] - [AR]} \quad (B.13)$$

Equating equations B.11 and B.13 and rearranging yields:

$$\text{Response} = \frac{[AR] \bullet E_m \bullet K_A}{[A](K_A - \nu) + [R_t]\nu} \quad (B.14)$$

If $K_A < \nu$ then negative and/or infinite values for response are allowed (no physiological counterpart to such behavior exists). Therefore this allows only a linear relationship between agonist concentration and response (where $K_A = \nu$) or a hyperbolic one ($K_A > \nu$). Very few cases of truly linear relationships between agonist concentration and tissue response can be found; therefore, the default for the relationship is a hyperbolic one.

A hyperbolic relationship between response and the amount of agonist–receptor complex, response is defined as:

$$\frac{\text{Response}}{E_{max}} = \frac{[AR]}{[AR] + K_E} \quad (B.15)$$

where K_E is the fitting parameter for the hyperbolic response. K_E has a pharmacological meaning in that it is the concentration of the [AR] complex that produces half the maximal response and it defines the ease with which the agonist produces response (i.e., it is a transduction constant). The more efficient the process from production of [AR] to response the smaller is K_E. Combining equations B.14 and B.15 yields the primary equation for the operational model:

$$Response = \frac{[A] \cdot [R_t] \cdot E_m}{[A]([R_t] + K_E) + K_A \cdot K_E} \quad (B.16)$$

A constant is defined that characterizes the propensity of a given system and a given agonist to yield response as the ratio $[R_t]/K_E$. This is denoted by τ. Substituting for τ yields the working equation for the operational model (equation 3.3):

$$Response = \frac{[A] \cdot \tau \cdot E_m}{[A](\tau + 1) + K_A} \quad (B.17)$$

B4 DERIVATION OF VARIABLE SLOPE BLACK–LEFF OPERATIONAL MODEL

For Chapter 3

If the stimulus–response coupling mechanism has inherent cooperativity, then a model with variable slope must be defined. The method for doing this involves re-expressing the receptor occupancy and/or activation expression (defined by the particular molecular model of receptor function) in terms of the operational model with Hill coefficient not equal to unity. The operational model utilizes the concentration of response-producing receptor as the substrate for a Michaelis–Menten type of reaction, given as:

$$Response = \frac{[Activated\ Receptor]E_m}{[Activated\ Receptor] + K_E} \quad (B.18)$$

where K_E is the concentration of activated receptor species that produces half-maximal response in the cell and E_{max} is the maximal capability of response production by the cell. Cooperativity expressed at the level of the cell can be expressed as a form of equation B.18 shown as:

$$Response = \frac{[Activated\ Receptor]^n E_m}{[Activated\ Receptor]^n + K_{E^n}} \quad (B.19)$$

where n is the slope of the concentration–response curve. The quantity of activated receptor is given by $\rho_{AR} \times [R_t]$, where ρ_{AR} is the fraction of total receptor in the activated form and $[R_t]$ is the total receptor density of the preparation. Substituting into equation B.19 and defining $\tau = [R_t]/K_E$ yields:

$$Response = \frac{\rho_{AR^n} \tau^n E_m}{\rho_{AR^n} \tau^n + 1} \quad (B.20)$$

The fractional receptor species ρ_{AR} is generally given by:

$$\rho_{AR^n} = \frac{[Active\ Receptor\ Species]^n}{[Total\ Receptor\ Species]^n} \quad (B.21)$$

where the active receptor species are the ones producing response and the total receptor species is given by the receptor conservation equation for the particular system (ρ_{AR} = numerator/denominator). It follows that:

$$Response$$
$$= \frac{(Active\ Receptor)^n \tau^n E_m}{(Active\ Receptor)^n \tau^n + (Total\ Receptor)^n} \quad (B.22)$$

Therefore, the operational model for agonism can be rewritten for variable slope by passing the stimulus equation through a forcing function to yield (see Fig. 3.5):

$$Response = \frac{\tau^n \cdot [A]^n \cdot E_m}{([A] + K_A)^n + \tau^n (A)^n} \quad (B.23)$$

B5 DERIVATION OF THE GADDUM EQUATION FOR COMPETITIVE ANTAGONISM

For Chapter 4

Analogous to competitive displacement binding, agonist [A] and antagonist [B] compete for receptor (R) occupancy:

$$
\begin{array}{c}
\text{B} \\
+ \\
\text{A} + \text{R} \xrightleftharpoons{K_a} \text{AR} \\
\Big\updownarrow K_b \\
\text{BR}
\end{array}
\tag{B.24}
$$

Where K_a and K_b are the respective ligand–receptor association constants.

The following equilibrium constants are defined:

$$[R] = \frac{[AR]}{[A]K_a} \tag{B.25}$$

$$[BR] = K_b[B][R] = \frac{K_b[B][AR]}{[A]K_a} \tag{B.26}$$

Total receptor concentration

$$[R_{tot}] = [R] + [AR] + [BR] \tag{B.27}$$

Leading to the expression for the response producing species $[AR]/[R_{tot}]$ (denoted as ρ):

$$\rho = \frac{[A]K_a}{[A]K_a + [B]K_b + 1} \tag{B.28}$$

Converting to equilibrium dissociation constants ($K_A = 1/K_a$) and redefining $[A]/K_A = c_A$ and $[B]/K_B = c_B$ leads to the Gaddum equation (equation 4.1):

$$\rho = \frac{c_A}{c_A + c_B + 1} \tag{B.29}$$

B6 CORRECTION OF IC$_{50}$ TO PK$_B$ FOR COMPETITIVE ANTAGONISTS

As shown by Leff and Dougall (Chapter 4; reference [3]) mass action equations can be used to derive the relationship between the concentration of antagonist that produces a 50% inhibition of a response to an agonist (antagonist concentration is referred to as the IC$_{50}$) and the equilibrium dissociation constant of the antagonist–receptor complex (K_B). The response in the absence of antagonist can be fit to a logistic curve of the form:

$$\text{Response} = \frac{E_m[A]^n}{[A]^n + [EC_{50}]^n} \tag{B.30}$$

where the concentration of agonist is [A], E_m is the maximal response to the agonist, n is the Hill coefficient of the dose–response curve and [EC$_{50}$] is the molar concentration of agonist producing 50% maximal response to the agonist.

In the presence of a competitive antagonist, the EC$_{50}$ of the agonist dose–response curve will shift to the right by a factor equal to the dose ratio; this is given by the Schild equation as $([B]/K_B + 1)$ where the concentration of the antagonist is [B] and K_B is the equilibrium dissociation constant of the antagonist–receptor complex:

$$\text{Response} = \frac{E_m[A']^n}{[A']^n + ([EC_{50}](1 + [B]/K_B))^n} \tag{B.31}$$

The concentration of antagonist producing a 50% diminution of the agonist response to concentration [A] is defined as the IC$_{50}$ for the antagonist. Therefore:

$$\frac{0.5E_{max}[A]^n}{[A]^n + [EC_{50}]^n} = \frac{E_m[A']^n}{[A']^n + ([EC_{50}](1 + [IC_{50}]/K_B))^n} \tag{B.32}$$

After rearrangement (equation 4.5):

$$K_B = \frac{[IC_{50}]}{((2 + ([A]/[EC_{50}])^n)^{1/n}) - 1} \tag{B.33}$$

B7 DERIVATION OF THE EQUATION FOR NON-COMPETITIVE ANTAGONISM

For Chapter 4

It is assumed that the non-competitive antagonist reduces the fraction of available receptor population. Assuming the non-competitive antagonist removes a fraction ρ_B from the receptor population, the fraction of agonist remaining after binding of B (ρ_{AB}) is given by:

$$\rho_{AB} = \frac{[A](1 - \rho_B)}{[A] + K_A} \qquad (B.34)$$

Expressing ρ_B from mass action:

$$(1 - \rho_B) = ([B]/K_B + 1) - 1 \qquad (B.35)$$

Equation B.35 can be rewritten for any slope value n:

$$\rho_{AB} = \frac{[A]^n}{([A] + K_A)^n ([B]/K_B + 1)^n} \qquad (B.36)$$

Substituting in B.20 yields (equation 4.6):

$$\text{Response} = \frac{[A]^n \tau^n E_m}{[A]^n \tau^n + (([A] + K_A)([B]/K_B + 1))^n} \qquad (B.37)$$

B8 DERIVATION OF THE EQUATION FOR ALLOSTERIC MODULATION

For Chapter 5

The equilibrium equations for the receptor species are:

$$[AR] = [ABR]/\alpha[B]K_b \qquad (B.38)$$

$$[BR] = [ABR]/\alpha[A]K_a \qquad (B.39)$$

$$[R] = [ABR]/\alpha[A]K_a[B]K_b \qquad (B.40)$$

The receptor conservation equation for total receptor $[R_{tot}]$ is:

$$[R_{tot}] = [R] + [AR] + [BR] + [ABR] \qquad (B.41)$$

The potential response producing species are [A] and [ABR]; therefore the fraction of receptors that may produce response is given by:

$$\rho_{A/B/AB} = \frac{[A]/K_A + \alpha[A]/K_A[B]/K_B}{[A]/K_A(1 + \alpha[B]/K_B) + [B]/K_B + 1} \qquad (B.42)$$

multiplying by $K_A K_B$ yields

$$\rho_{A/B/AB} = \frac{[A]K_B + \alpha[A][B]}{[A]K_B + \alpha[A][B] + [B]K_A + K_A K_B} \qquad (B.43)$$

From B.20:

$$\text{Response} = \frac{(\tau_A[A](K_B + \alpha[A][B]))^n E_m}{(\tau_A[A](K_B + \alpha[A][B]))^n + ([A]K_B + \alpha[A][B] + [B]K_A + K_A K_B)^n} \qquad (B.44)$$

Defining τ_B as $= \beta\tau_A$ gives (equation 5.2):

$$\text{Response} = \frac{(\tau_A[A](K_B + \alpha\beta[B]))^n E_m}{(\tau_A[A](K_B + \alpha\beta[B]))^n + ([A]K_B + K_A K_B + K_A[B] + \alpha[A][B])^n} \qquad (B.45)$$

B9 DERIVATION OF THE EQUATION FOR ALLOSTERIC MODULATION WITH DIRECT AGONISM

In this case, the modulator occupied receptor can also produce response due to direct efficacy. Therefore, the potential response producing species are [A], [BR] and [ABR]; therefore the fraction of receptors that may produce response is given by:

$$\rho_{A/B/AB} = \frac{[A]/K_A + [B]/K_B + \alpha[A]/K_A[B]/K_B}{[A]/K_A(1 + \alpha[B]/K_B) + [B]/K_B + 1} \qquad (B.46)$$

$$\rho_{A/B/AB} = \frac{[A]/K_B + [B]/K_A + \alpha[A][B]}{[A]K_B + \alpha[A][B] + [B]K_A + K_A K_B}$$

(B.47)

From B.20

$$\text{Response} = \frac{(\tau_A[A](K_B + \alpha[A][B]) + \tau_B[B]K_A)^n E_m}{(\tau_A[A](K_B + \alpha[A][B]) + \tau_B[B]K_A)^n + ([A]K_B + \alpha[A][B] + [B]K_A + K_A K_B)^n}$$

(B.48)

Defining τ_B as $= \beta\tau_A$ gives (equation 5.3):

$$\text{Response} = \frac{(\tau_A[A](K_B + \alpha\beta[B]) + \tau_B[B]K_A)^n E_m}{(\tau_A[A](K_B + \alpha\beta[B]) + \tau_B[B]K_A)^n + ([A]K_B + K_A K_B + K_A[B] + \alpha[A][B])^n}$$

(B.49)

B10 DERIVATION OF THE MICHAELIS−MENTEN EQUATION FOR ENZYMES

For Chapter 6

The reaction scheme for Michaelis-Menten kinetics is:

$$E + S \underset{k_{-1}}{\overset{k_1}{\rightleftharpoons}} ES \overset{k_2}{\longrightarrow} E + P$$

(B.50)

The substrate binds reversibly to the enzyme to form a complex ES which either dissociates or progresses to enzyme plus a product P. The product P is assumed to have no affinity for the enzyme and thus dissociates. The second half of the reaction describes an irreversible formation of product plus regeneration of the active enzyme. From the reaction scheme B.50 comes an expression for the velocity ν for the enzyme reaction:

$$\nu = k_2[ES]$$

(B.51)

The assumption here is that the overall reaction velocity is limited by the formation of product. At this point the assumption is made that the amount of ES complex is nearly constant such that the rate of formation of ES

(controlled by rate constant k_1) is equal to the rates of dissociation going forward (k_2) and backward (k_{-1}):

$$k_1[E][S] = k_{-1}[ES] + k_2[ES]$$

(B.52)

Which rearranges to:

$$\frac{k_1[E][S]}{(k_{-1} + k_2)} = [ES]$$

(B.53)

A rate constant K_m (the Michaelis−Menten constant) is defined:

$$\frac{(k_{-1} + k_2)}{k_1} = K_M$$

(B.54)

which allows equation B.53 to be written:

$$\frac{[E][S]}{K_M} = [ES]$$

(B.55)

The total enzyme concentration $[E_0]$ is given by the conservation equation:

$$[E_0] = [E] + [ES]$$

(B.56)

Solving for [E] and substituting into B.55 yields:

$$\frac{([E_0] - [ES]) + [S]}{K_M} = [ES]$$

(B.57)

Rearrangement of B.57 and solving for [ES] yields:

$$\frac{[E_0][S]}{[S] + K_M} = [ES]$$

(B.58)

Substituting equation B.58 into equation B.51 yields:

$$\nu = k_2 \frac{[E_0][S]}{[S] + K_M} \tag{B.59}$$

Defining a maximal rate of enzyme reaction V_{max} which occurs when $[S] \gg [E]$ (also defined as $[A] \rightarrow \infty$) yields:

$$v_{max} = k_2[E_0] \tag{B.60}$$

Substituting equation B.60 into equation B.59 yields the Michaelis–Menten equation:

$$\nu = \frac{V_{max}[S]}{K_M + [S]} \tag{B.61}$$

Index

Printed and bound by CPI Group (UK) Ltd, Croydon, CR0 4YY

08/06/2025

01896872-0016